LIVE ANOTHER

4006 DAYS

AND IMPROVE YOUR

HEALTH

With DENTAL MEDICINE

RICHARD GUYVER

LIVE ANOTHER
4006
DAYS
AND IMPROVE YOUR
HEALTH
With DENTAL
MEDICINE

THE
ULTIMATE
Guide to UNDERSTANDING the Link between
ORAL HEALTH and
GENERAL HEALTH

Advantage®

Published by Advantage, Charleston, South Carolina.
Member of Advantage Media Group.

ADVANTAGE is a registered trademark and the Advantage colophon is a trademark of Advantage Media Group, Inc.

Printed in the United States of America.

ISBN: 978-159932-404-3
LCCN: 2013939203

This publication is designed to provide accurate and authoritative information in regard to the subject matter covered. It is sold with the understanding that the publisher is not engaged in rendering legal, accounting, or other professional services. If legal advice or other expert assistance is required, the services of a competent professional person should be sought.

Advantage Media Group is proud to be a part of the Tree Neutral® program. Tree Neutral offsets the number of trees consumed in the production and printing of this book by taking proactive steps such as planting trees in direct proportion to the number of trees used to print books. To learn more about Tree Neutral, please visit www.treeneutral.com. To learn more about Advantage's commitment to being a responsible steward of the environment, please visit www.advantagefamily.com/green

Advantage Media Group is a publisher of business, self-improvement, and professional development books and online learning. We help entrepreneurs, business leaders, and professionals share their Stories, Passion, and Knowledge to help others Learn & Grow™. Do you have a manuscript or book idea that you would like us to consider for publishing? Please visit advantagefamily.com or call 1.866.775.1696.

Contents

> *WARNING: This section should not be read by dentists who act unethically or who do not want to provide up-to-date care for their patients*

List of images

IMAGE 1

Dental Medicine Triangle: shows the three cornerstones behind the philosophy of Dental Medicine

IMAGE 2

The marginal ridge of the tooth, loss of the marginal ridge through decay will significantly affect the ridgity of the tooth

IMAGE 3

An overhanging filling which is impossible to clean effectively

IMAGE 4

An x-ray picture of the tooth in image 3 showing the challenge that such a poorly placed restoration creates for effective cleaning

IMAGE 5

A draining infection from a tooth which gave no apparent pain or symptoms

IMAGE 6

An x-ray picture of the tooth from image 5 showing the infection at the top of the root

IMAGE 7

An x-ray picture of the tooth from images 5 and 6 showing the root canal filling in the tooth root

IMAGE 8

A photo of the same tooth from images 5, 6 and 7 showing the draining infection has now resolved following appropriate treatment

IMAGE 9

An indication of the mechanisms of how inflammation can impact on diabetes and glycaemic control

IMAGE 10

A diagram to show atheromatous (arterial) diseases and the conditions it can cause

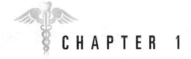

CHAPTER 1

Dental Medicine

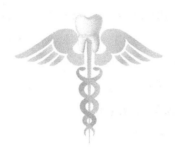

Congratulations on choosing to read a book that will help you to discover what you can do to improve both your oral health and your general health. My aim is to be able to help you have a long and healthy life. I can help you gain the knowledge to ensure you are doing what is best for your health, and to know the right questions to ask your dental team. You will hold the power to enable you to achieve the outcome you desire. With that power, I estimate you could live an extra 4006 days. How have I calculated that you could live an extra 4006 days? The calculation and explanation appears in Chapter 26.

You may be wondering what the benefits of reading this book are. Well here's a list of some of them:

- live a longer life
- live a healthier life
- improve your oral health
- require less medical intervention

- require less dental intervention
- save money on your dental care
- learn some tips on things you can do yourself
- take greater control over your health
- decide if a particular dental team is the right team for you

Just think, by taking some steps now, you could increase the time you have to spend with your loved ones. You could now get the chance to do some of those things that are really life changing; perhaps take the trip of a lifetime. We all wonder if we will be healthy, particularly as we clock up the years. Now you can stop wondering and start to take control. I am always astounded at how far medical research has come over the last twenty years. The things we know now mean that it is more realistic for us to take control of our health, and ensure we are doing everything we can for our own future. The barrier is often knowledge, or more specifically, lack of appropriate knowledge and how to use it. Much of the research stays locked away in medical journals and is only accessible by those of us who have access to those journals. Much of the research is written in medical jargon, and as such is inaccessible to members of the public even if they can get access to those journals. Then there is the conflict; some research proves one thing; other research disproves it. Someone needs to be able to separate out the good studies so we can reach meaningful conclusions.

What I have tried to do in this book is to take the medical research around oral health and turn it into something from which you can benefit. You will not find pages of information on how studies were carried out. You will not find tables and graphs of data, or extensive statistical analyses. To be frank, most people would not read them, and I think we should leave all that to the academics. This book is a bridge between that academic world and real life.

This is not a medical text book. It's a book for you, a member of the public, who wants to be sure that you are doing all that you can to have a long and healthy life. It is aimed at three groups of people

1. Those with an existing medical condition who want to be sure that their mouth is not worsening that disease
2. Those who want to avoid getting any of a number of medical conditions
3. It is also useful for professionals, particularly dental teams who want to be sure they can provide the best care possible for their patients

The real benefit in reading this book is that it will empower you to ask your doctor/dentist the right questions. It will also give you an insight into the benefits of certain interventions which not only help your mouth but also your general health. It's not possible to write a book such as this without using a little medical terminology, so I apologise in advance. Hopefully the explanations that go with the technical terms will be of use to you. (There is a glossary at the end which defines various terms I use through the book.) You will also find references to the images, all images will be found in the centre of the book.

There are additional resources that are available to readers of this book. Go to www.4006days.com; you will need the following code to access the resources (not case sensitive): hgy4006jujth

Dental Medicine is the study of how the mouth (i.e. oral health) has an impact on the body (i.e. general health), and vice versa. We are also interested in how the intervention by dentists (or indeed the lack of intervention) impacts on both oral and general health. There are three interrelated principles:

1. The impact of the body on the mouth
2. The impact of the mouth on the body
3. The ability to use the mouth to help identify medical concerns

These three cornerstones make up the Dental Medicine Triangle, see Image 1.

So Dental Medicine is also a philosophy of care, a philosophy in which we view our patients as whole people. Every action we take (or do not take) will affect your general health and well-being. Dental Medicine Experts are very aware of this and will ensure that these actions and decisions will have a positive impact, and we make sure that you are aware of these impacts.

Those who are experts in Dental Medicine and who subscribe to its philosophy in their working practice pay special attention to the interaction of the three cornerstones as seen in image 1. This means we can help identify medical conditions and help reduce their impact on your mouth. We can positively improve general health by ensuring that there are no 'hidden killers' lurking in your mouth that are going to trigger a medical condition, or worsen your general health. All Dental Medicine Experts are dentists, but not all dentists are Dental Medicine Experts.

The Mouth Is a Window to the Body

Using the Mouth to Identify Medical Conditions

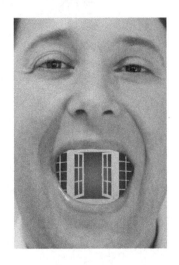

You may know that the mouth can be used as an indication that things are amiss elsewhere with your general health. At dental school, students are taught that the 'mouth is a window to the body'. The soft tissues (tongue, cheeks, gums, and so on) have a very rapid turnover which means that the building blocks which make up the tissues are rapidly renewed. If something goes awry which affects these building blocks (cells), an indication can often be seen, or felt, in the mouth.

The gums and teeth can also indicate that there is a problem somewhere. The list of conditions that can lead to a change such as this in the mouth include gastrointestinal diseases, diabetes, vitamin and mineral deficiencies, and certain dermatological (skin) conditions, to name a few.

I have dedicated a large part of this book to this area of Dental Medicine. Most of the signs that can be identified are most likely to be detected by an observant dental professional. An expert in Dental Medicine will be on the lookout for these signs every time he or she looks in your mouth. In this book I describe the symptoms that you may be aware of and what to do if you notice them.

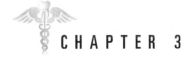

CHAPTER 3

General Health Can Have an Impact on the Mouth

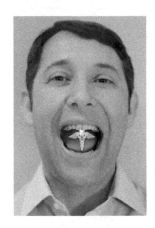

There is a long list of conditions that can have a harmful impact on your mouth, and an impact on what dentists do. It includes a comprehensive list of drugs, gastrointestinal diseases, diabetes, heart disease, osteoporosis, haematological (blood) conditions, and dermatological (skin) conditions. Most people will make lifestyle choices whilst taking into account their general health. It is unlikely that these choices will be significantly influenced by the knowledge that the choice could also have a positive effect on your oral health. It makes sense to do what you can to stay healthy and so we will not really focus on this area in this book.

What you will find is that a dentist who is an expert in Dental Medicine will ask you about your general health as well as your mouth. This is because your general health will impact on what we do. In fact, all dentists should be asking these questions.

CHAPTER 4

Health Issues can be Triggered by the Mouth

So we have briefly seen that the mouth can be used to help us identify that there are certain health issues, and certain health issues can impact on the mouth. In my experience the real eye-opener comes when people realise that the mouth also has an impact on general health. This is so important that it is worth repeating: **the mouth also has an impact on general health.** This is the area that really excites experts in Dental Medicine. Of course we enjoy looking after people's mouths and giving them great teeth that increase their confidence and their comfort. Knowing that we can also reduce the risk of disease, help reduce the impact of existing disease and so have a positive impact on our patients' lifespan and quality of life is why we put ourselves through the extra training and study that is needed to be able to call ourselves Dental Medicine Experts. What could be more rewarding than helping a patient out, perhaps by identifying gum disease which they didn't know they had, helping them bring it under control and seeing, for example, their diabetes control improve? Or hearing that their doctor has reduced their blood pressure medication when they had been struggling with trying to control their blood pressure for many years before coming to us?

This is the area of Dental Medicine that I really focus on in this book. Dental Medicine Experts are passionate about improving their patients' health and quality of life. I wrote this book to share with you how we can do this and so you can find out what you can do.

HOW DOES THE MOUTH IMPACT GENERAL HEALTH?

This is one of the areas where I need to use some medical terminology. In most cases it is linked to inflammation. There are a number of potential causes of inflammation in the mouth. Inflammation is normally our friend, as it helps us to fight cuts, scrapes, and infections. However, when that inflammation carries on for a long time and becomes chronic inflammation, it can end up doing more harm than good.

There are a few theories as to how the mouth can have a detrimental impact on general health. It is likely that the evidence supporting one of them will increase over time, or even that we find out that more than mechanism is responsible.

The most likely theory, which is gaining more and more evidence and support, is as follows. Inflammation (e.g. in the mouth) will cause what is referred to as a pro-inflammatory state in the body. This means the body starts to release a number of so-called mediators (tiny messengers that help parts of the body tell other parts what is going on) into the blood stream. Think of nerves as the emails you send, and mediators as the letters you post.

It is the effect of these mediators, either directly or indirectly, that impacts on general health. One culprit is a protein called C-reactive protein (CRP) that is released into your blood when your body detects inflammation. CRP is used by doctors as an inflammation marker. This is a way that your body communicates that it is fighting inflammation. You often will not know that inflammation is going on. For example, with gum disease you often get no symptoms at all, or perhaps a little bit of bleeding when cleaning. This is not normal. If your scalp bled when you brushed your hair, it would (quite rightly) cause alarm. The same is true of gums.

QUICK FACTS: BLEEDING GUMS

Bleeding gums are normally due to inflammation and rarely due to overzealous oral hygiene techniques.

The liver produces CRP, but not all the time. In healthy people it may not even show up in a blood test. When the body starts to develop inflammation, it releases a number of mediators, each of which has its own specific role. Some of these mediators tell the liver to start releasing CRP.

WHY DO WE HAVE CRP AND MEDIATORS?

The mediators are set loose at the area where there is a problem (be it an injury or infection) and tell the rest of the body what is happening. This tends to start a chain of events, the ultimate aim being to correct the problem.

The role of CRP is to detect and identify dead or dying cells. It effectively 'paints a target' on them. This targeted cell is then detected by other parts of the immune system which destroys those cells.

IT'S NOT ALL GOOD NEWS

CRP and other mediators, however, can have a detrimental effect, particularly if they are allowed to hang around for long periods of time. They have been shown to lead to increased risk of certain conditions including diabetes, cardiovascular disease, strokes, high blood pressure and possibly even Alzheimer's disease. The list of conditions linked to such mediators seems to grow each year and will probably continue to do so.

IT'S NOT ALL BAD NEWS EITHER

We have seen that there are links between inflammation and mediators such as CRP. There is also a link between CRP and medical conditions. The good news is that removing inflammation (e.g. through treating gum disease) will decrease the levels of CRP and therefore help reduce the risk of getting these diseases. Studies show that by treating gum disease successfully, or by removing oral inflammation, patients were significantly more likely to have a reduction in C-reactive protein levels.[1]

---

1   Mattila, K. et al., 'Effect of Treating Periodontitis on C-reactive Protein Levels: A Pilot Study', *BMC Infect. Dis.*, 2 (2002), 30.

Chen, L. et al., 'Effects of Non-surgical Periodontal Treatment on Clinical Response, Serum Inflammatory Parameters, and Metabolic Control in Type 2 Diabetes: A Randomized Study', *J. Periodontol.*, 83/4 (April 2012), DOI: 10.1902/jop.2011.110327, 435–43.

Taylor, B. A. et al., 'Full Mouth Tooth Extraction Lowers Systemic Inflammatory and Thrombotic Markers of Cardiovascular Disease', *J. Dent Res.*, 85/1 (2006), 74–8.

Paraskevas, S., Huizinga, J. D., and Loos, B. G., 'A Systematic Review and Meta-Analysis on C-reactive Protein in Relation to Periodontitis', *J. Clin. Periodontol.*, 35/4 (2008), 277–90.

CHAPTER 5

The Multifactorial Nature of Disease

n reality, it is likely that all diseases are multifactorial. This means that there have to be a number of 'factors' occurring before someone will get the disease. This is why we hear stories from people about someone they know, perhaps an elderly relative who smoked sixty a day for sixty years and died at the ripe old age of ninety! This happens not because smoking actually causes a disease such as lung cancer, but because it is one of the factors that increase the likelihood of getting such a disease.

If you, without looking, crossed a quiet country road that sees very little traffic, it is unlikely that you would get hit by a car, but it may happen. If you were to do the same on a busy motorway, the chance of you getting hit would be much higher. However, you may be lucky and not get hit. If you were to do this sixty times a day, the likelihood of getting hit increases in both scenarios. It is unlikely that you would see the day out crossing the M40 sixty times a day without looking; on the quiet country road you may still be OK. It's all down to probability and chance. Triggers for diseases are exactly the same. Just because you have one of the risk factors does not mean you will get the disease. In the same way, not possessing the risk factor will not mean that you will not get the disease (sorry for the use of a triple negative there!) It simply affects the risk. The more risk factors you have, the higher the risk, or the more you are exposed to risk factors, the higher the risk.

So inflammation in the mouth is one of the risk factors for a number of diseases. As you will find out from reading this book, it is one of the significant factors. However, all diseases are likely to be multifactorial. Those with inflammation are crossing a busier road than those without, so are more likely to get hit.

The prevention message is, therefore, that we should aim to reduce/eliminate as many of the risk factors as we can in order for you to enjoy a long healthy life. We all have to cross the road; let's make sure we can do it the least number of times and the safest way possible!

Be sure to read about all the medical conditions, even if you think you are not susceptible. You may be surprised by what you find out!

CHAPTER 6

What Role Can Oral Health Play?

Wear and tear on teeth is expected. After all, we are living longer and our teeth are not really designed to work for as long as they have to! Typical life expectancy 2000 years ago was about twenty-one years. As time goes on, our teeth need more and more care to keep then functioning well and looking good. Just like an old car, after forty years of use, we expect that it will need some replacement parts, and regular oil changes, new brake pads, and so on. The teeth and the mouth are no different. Keeping with the car metaphor, carrying out this maintenance means we are less likely to have a breakdown. Most cars spend a great deal of their time sitting idle; our mouths are on the go twenty-four hours a day. By the time you are sixty years old, you mouth has clocked up over half a million working hours! If you consider the harsh environment which our mouths (including teeth and restorations) are subject to, it's hardly surprising that some intervention is needed. Harsh factors that our mouths are subject to include the following:

- hot foods and drinks, such as tea and coffee
- cold foods and drinks, such as ice cream
- biting forces that can exert hundreds of pounds of pressure thousands of times a day

- an environment which changes from being acidic to non-acidic throughout the day
- an environment which changes from being dry to being bathed in liquid
- a constant onslaught from bacteria and the toxic substances which they produce
- any habits such as nail biting will further increase the wear and tear

If there is already a restoration in the tooth, which is then subject to this onslaught, it's not surprising that we need to intervene. There's a part of the back teeth (the molars and premolars) called the marginal ridge. This is the part of the tooth which touches the next door tooth, see Image 2. If there is a restoration already in this area (i.e. if the marginal ridge has been lost) on just one side of the tooth the rigidity of that tooth is decreased by 46%. If both marginal ridges are lost then the rigidity is decreased by a massive 63%.[2] So if we could have prevented that decay in the first place (or helped it to reverse back to healthy tooth by identifying it early and introducing an appropriate prevention package) then your tooth could potentially have avoided losing two thirds of its rigidity! The benefits of prevention are accepted by all, however the actual numbers of dentists practicing these methods remains surprisingly low.

A tooth that has lost 63% of its rigidity and is subject to the wear and tear outlined above will need multiple restorations over its life. Each one will be slightly larger than the previous one. How much money could you save over the lifetime of a tooth if you could

---

2 Monga P., Sharma V. and Kumar S., 'Comparison of fracture resistance of endodontically treated teeth using different coronal restorative materials: An in vitro study', *J. Conserv. Dent.*, 12/4 (2009), 154-159.

avoid needing the restoration in the first place? In view of all this it may not surprise you to find out that dentists detect things in the mouth that are not ideal. The scary thing is that they are compromising not just your oral health but your general health and therefore lifespan and quality of life.

SIGNS THAT YOU OR YOUR DENTIST MAY SEE

There are some things that you may notice and others that your dentist may notice.

By ensuring you do not have these signs (by making sure your mouth is healthy and free from inflammation), we can reduce your risk of getting diabetes, heart disease, stroke, chronic lung disease, low-birth-weight/premature babies, certain cancers, and dementia.

BLEEDING AND GUM DISEASE

Most people have low-grade infections in their mouths all the time. You may have noticed blood on a toothbrush, floss, or when spitting out after cleaning. If your dentist carries out a gum assessment, he or she will detect if there is any bleeding. This bleeding only occurs when there is inflammation, and as we now know, there are established links between inflammation and general health.

Smoking can mask this bleeding as it decreases the blood flow to the gums and supporting bone. That means there can be inflammation present that does not show up, which is even worse as it is more likely to be missed.

CRACKS AND TOOTH WEAR

Any crack in a tooth which goes beyond the gum will lead to localised gum inflammation. A crack of 0.1 mm will be like a twenty-lane superhighway for bacteria, often leaving you with no hope of being able to clean it out. It's more likely that a dentist will pick up these cracks, although you may see them on some teeth. It is not always necessary to treat them if they are not causing gum inflammation.

Excessive tooth wear may be a sign that your teeth are not 'up to the job' of chewing, and as we will see, not being able to chew effectively can have far-reaching effects.

DECAY

Decay is essentially a collection of bacteria which actively causes inflammation. So, any decay should be eliminated as soon as possible.

VOIDS OR OVERHANGING FILLINGS/CROWNS

A filling or crown that has not been made or fitted very well or has worn away over time will lead to an area where bacteria can exist and thrive. This, in turn will lead to inflammation.

Image 3 shows a photograph of a tooth with an overhang, and Image 4, the corresponding X-ray picture. This demonstrates an area that is impossible to clean.

DRY MOUTH

Experiencing a dry mouth can be unpleasant. Saliva carries immune components which help the body destroy bacteria. So having less saliva decreases the effectiveness of this process and increases the risk of decay.

FUNGAL INFECTIONS

Our mouths are teeming with billions of little bugs; more than 700 different types have been identified. They are a combination of bacteria and fungi. Normally these live in harmony, and our immune system keeps a check on them, so no one species can take over. Every so often something can interrupt this balance and some take over. It tends to be the fungi, and this can lead to thrush or other fungal infections. When this happens, it leads to inflammation. Some fungal infections (particularly in patients whose immune system is not functioning well) can be so severe that they can destroy the underlying bone. When I worked in hospital in the maxillofacial surgery department, I treated a patient who lost his entire top jaw due to a fungal infection.

HIDDEN INFECTIONS

QUICK FACTS: LUMPS ON THE GUM

Don't ignore that blister/lump on the gum, even if it is not painful. Often these little lumps appear when there is an infection from a tooth and mean there is inflammation present.

It is possible to have an infection from a tooth which gives either no symptoms or such mild symptoms that they are passed off as normal. These hidden infections are causing inflammation all the time. Sometimes we pick them up on X-ray pictures, sometimes from a small bubble that appears on the gum overlying the root. Unfortunately, a lot of dentists do not treat these as they are not painful. However, they are likely to have a negative impact on your general health.

Image 5 shows a photograph of a hidden infection, and the corresponding X-ray picture in Image 6. The X-ray picture shows some early changes in the bone around the top of the root caused by the infection. The patient did not know she had an on-going infection here. The infection was caused as the nerve in the tooth had died. The nerve lives in a tunnel in the tooth. When it dies, the tunnel fills with bacteria and it is these bacteria that cause the infection.

After successful root canal treatment the X-ray picture (Image 7) shows the root filling and the photograph (Image 8) shows that the small swelling on the gum has disappeared, indicating that the infection has been eliminated.

QUICK FACTS:

SIGNS OF INFLAMMATION THAT A DENTIST SHOULD LOOK FOR:

- bleeding
- gum disease

- cracks in teeth
- decay
- voids or overhangs in restorations
- dry mouth
- fungal infections
- hidden infections
- smoking

SMOKING AND TOBACCO: A SPECIAL CONCERN

Smoking decreases your body's ability to fight gum inflammation, which worsens the risk of suffering from gum disease. Smoking can have an indirect impact on many of the diseases in this book that are related to inflammation. It also hides the early warning signs of gum inflammation so it may be that gum disease, for example, is more established by the time it can be detected.

Smoking is also a direct 'risk factor' for a number of diseases including diabetes, heart disease, lung disease, cancer, impotence, pregnancy complications, and stroke. In fact, smoking seems to have a direct impact on the risk of many of the diseases that are also affected by the mouth!

Although not strictly a 'disease', tobacco influences many of the other diseases that we have mentioned earlier, so it earns its own place in this book.

ROLE OF DENTAL MEDICINE IN TOBACCO USE

Those who use tobacco require close monitoring as they are at increased risk of many oral and non-oral diseases.

We also take an active role in smoking cessation for those who want to stop. If you are a smoker and keen to stop, a Dental Medicine Expert will be able to help and point you in the right direction.

CHAPTER 7

Medical Conditions and Diseases That Dental Medicine Experts Can Directly Influence

I n the next stage of the book I will describe a number of medical conditions and their link with the mouth. You will also find some sections that are not strictly 'medical conditions', but are things that are worth considering. First I will look at diet, nutrition, and chewing ability.

For each disease I will give a bit of background to the disease itself and then introduce the way it impacts on our mouths, and the way our mouths impact on it.

SPECIAL CASES: VICIOUS CIRCLES!

Among the conditions that we will be looking at in this book, these are especially important. They are the ones in which the mouth can impact directly on the disease, AND the disease impact on the mouth. This creates a vicious circle and until the cycle is broken, deterioration of both the mouth and general health continues.

Look for this symbol to see the relevant diseases where a vicious circle exists:

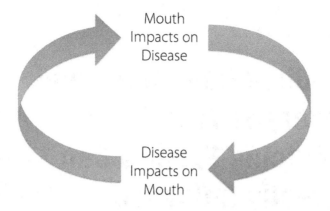

CHAPTER 8

Diet, Nutrition, and Chewing Ability

We know that our diet plays a role in our general health. We all hear the news stories that state a certain food is good for you, a certain food is bad for you. I would expect over the next ten years or so that we will see an increased recognition in the role that diet and nutrition play in our general health.

In chapter 14 'Dementia and Alzheimer's Disease' we will see that those who struggle with chewing are more likely to develop dementia.[3] One challenge that people have if they cannot chew properly (perhaps as they are missing teeth, have dentures that rub, or gum disease that means their teeth are not firm) is they cannot eat the healthier kinds of foods, or they need to cook them so much that the nutrients are removed. They tend to eat processed foods which are unhealthier and higher in sugar content. They avoid those foods which are healthier and protective.[4] If you struggle with eating a

3   Paganini-Hill, A., White, S. C., and Atchison, K. A., 'Dentition, Dental Habits and Dementia: The Leisure World Cohort Study', *J. Am. Ger. Soc.,* 60/8 (2012), 1556-63.

Lexomboom, D., Trulsson, M., Wardh, I., and Parker, M. G., 'Chewing Ability and Tooth Loss: Associated with Cognitive Impairment in an Elderley Population Study', *J. Am. Geriatr. Soc.,* 60/10 (2012), 1951-6.

4   Glynn, Sarah, 'Green Veggies Reduce the Risk of Oral Cancer', Medical News Today (4 Oct. 2012) <http://www.medicalnewstoday.com/articles/251153.php>.

balanced diet which includes healthy food such as vegetables, perhaps it's worth speaking to your dentist to see what can be done to help.

Below, I look at some specific vitamins and minerals and their links with oral health.

INTERESTING FACTS: COFFEE

Coffee used to be thought of as a 'bad' drink. However, recent research shows that coffee has a protective role.

COFFEE AND CANCER

There is some evidence that oral cancer risk can be reduced. Those who drink four cups of caffeinated coffee a day have a 49% lower risk of death from oral cancer.[5]

COFFEE AND DIABETES

Coffee helps protect against type 2 diabetes. There is a lot of evidence that regular coffee intake reduces the risk of getting diabetes, with each additional cup (up to eight cups a day) being associated with a 5–10% lower risk.[6] The exact mechanism of protection is not yet known. However, it does not appear to be related to caffeine.

---

5 Hildebrand, J. S., 'Coffee, Tea, and Fatal Oral/Pharyngeal Cancer in a Large Prospective U.S. Cohort', *Am. J. Epidemiol.*, 177/1 (2013), 50–8.

6 Huxley, R. et al., 'Decaffeinated Coffee, and Tea Consumption in Relation to Incident Type 2 Diabetes Mellitus', *Arch. Intern. Med.*, 169/22 (2009), 2053–63.

129. van Dam, R. M. et al., 'Coffee Consumption and Risk of Type 2 Diabetes Mellitus', Lancet, 360/9344 (2002), 1477–8.

COFFEE AND OTHER CONDITIONS

Coffee may also play a protective role against prostate cancer,[7] Alzheimer's disease and dementia,[8] Parkinson's disease, heart disease, fatty liver disease,[9] and cirrhosis.[10]

VITAMINS AND MINERALS

Your mouth can often give the first signs and symptoms of vitamin and mineral deficiencies. The main nutrients that can affect it are vitamin B12, folic acid, and iron. Soreness of the tongue, ulcers in the mouth, redness or sore spots developing at the corners of the mouth, the tongue becoming smoother, or fungal infections like oral thrush can all be indicators that there is a deficiency. If you, or your dentist, identifies these signs, it may be worth seeing your doctor for some blood tests to help establish the cause.

Vitamin and mineral deficiencies can contribute to other conditions such as cancer and a weakened immune system.

Another indication of the connection between nutrition and oral health: vitamin D given to children (or produced by them, as

---

7   Wilson, K. M. et al., 'Coffee Consumption and Prostate Cancer Risk and Progression in the Health Professionals Follow-up Study', *J. Natl. Cancer Inst.*, 103/11 (2011), 876–84.

8   Eskelinen, M. et al., 'Midlife Coffee and Tea Drinking and the Risk of Late-Life Dementia: A Population-Based CAIDE Study', *J. Alzheimer's Dis.*, 16/1 (2009), 85–91.

9   Catalano, D. et al., 'Protective Role of Coffee in Non-alcoholic Fatty Liver Disease', *Dig. Dis. Sci.*, 55/11 (2010), 3200–6.

10   Klatsky, A. L. et al., 'Coffee, Cirrhosis, and Transaminase Enzymes', *Arch. Intern. Med.*, 166/11 (2006), 1190–5.

UV radiation from the sun causes vitamin D to be produced) has been shown to reduce the risk of dental decay by as much as 50%.[11]

ROLE OF DENTAL MEDICINE IN DIET AND CHEWING ABILITY

Our role in encouraging and promoting great general health means Dental Medicine Experts will be keen to ensure that their patients' ability to eat a balanced diet is not being prevented by their mouth. We would always want to provide a set of teeth that allow you to eat a healthy diet.

The connection between good nutrition and a lowered risk of a variety of medical conditions and diseases is well established. If you cannot eat or chew properly, you are being let down by your mouth, and there will be an impact on your general health. A Dental Medicine Expert will always be on the lookout for the early warning signs of a vitamin/mineral deficiency so that intervention can start as soon as possible, thereby reducing the likelihood of any long-term damage.

---

11 Hujoel, P. P., 'Vitamin D and Dental Caries in Controlled Clinical Trials: Systematic Review and Meta-Analysis', *Nutrition Reviews*, 21/2 (2012), 88-97.

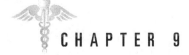

CHAPTER 9

Diabetes

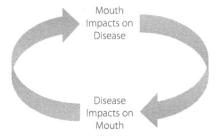

Mouth Impacts on Disease

Disease Impacts on Mouth

There is a very good reason why diabetes is the first disease I address. Diabetes appears in all three corners of our Dental Medicine Triangle as seen in image 1. Due to this, it is one of the important medical conditions that Dental Medicine Experts take into consideration. This is not because the others are less important, but diabetes is the one where we can have the most influence. As it happens, the principles we teach dentists so they can manage diabetes and the mouth are applicable to all of the other medical conditions that we need to consider. The training of dentists to become experts in Dental Medicine is carried out by the Diabetes and Dentistry Organisation (www.diabetesanddentistry.co.uk) which is affiliated with the Dental Medicine Academy (www.dentalmedicine.co.uk). Diabetes is also the condition on which much of the research has been based when looking at the impact of the mouth on disease.

WHAT IS DIABETES?

When we eat food and that food is broken down in the gut, it releases sugars. Those sugars are absorbed into the blood stream. In order for our body to be able to use those sugars, they need to be allowed to enter our cells. However, the door is locked and the key to open that door is called insulin. Without insulin the door stays firmly closed and sugar does not enter the cells. This means that surplus sugars are floating around in the blood stream. It is this which causes damage to organs. In diabetes either there is no insulin produced, or the amount of insulin is too low, or the insulin is not effective (i.e. the key doesn't fit the lock any more).

Diabetes affects around 2.8 million people in the UK, with a further estimated 850,000 undiagnosed. It can lead to heart disease, higher risk of stroke, kidney failure, blindness, and amputation of limbs. Thousands of people die each year as a result of diabetes and its effects.

High blood-sugar levels can lead to a build-up of plaques on the lining of arteries (called atherosclerosis). These plaques cause inflammation which also releases CRP. This has been suggested as one of the reasons why those with diabetes are more likely to get the conditions, such as arterial disease, that are linked to high CRP.

About 10% of the UK National Health Service (NHS) budget (approximately £14 billion per year) is spent managing diabetes and it complications. In addition is the cost to the economy of lost work days, and early retirement and social benefits (estimated to be another £15–16 billion each year). The other cost, which is harder to quantify, is the cost of living with a chronic disease, its side effects, and the risk of a premature death.

As the prevalence of diabetes is increasing rapidly, these costs are likely to increase as well.

DIABETES MYTHS AND FACTS

It's worth dispelling some myths about diabetes at this stage.

Fact: we tend to look at diabetes as two types: type 1 and type 2

Fact: We do not know what causes type 1 diabetes (although there is a genetic role), but in type 1 the pancreas stops producing insulin, so the patient with type 1 has to get his or her insulin in a different way. Normally this is achieved through regular injections, or a small pump which is placed under the skin.

Myth: Type 2 diabetes is a milder form of diabetes. This is not true. Both are significant diseases which need to be well managed.

Myth: You get type 2 diabetes from eating too much sugar. This is not true. Diet does play a role, but it is the whole diet, not just sugar. Remember, all diseases are multifactorial. Diet is one of the factors.

Myth: Diabetes is not that serious. This is not true. It has a significant impact on peoples' lives, their overall health and their risk of an early death.

Myth: Type 2 diabetes only affects overweight people. This is also untrue. Many people who develop type 2 diabetes are not at all overweight. It is one of the risk factors, so being overweight increases the risk of developing type 2 diabetes.

Myth: Type 2 diabetes only affects older people. This is not true, and we are seeing an increasing number of young adults in their mid-20s developing the condition.

Myth: Diabetes leads to early death. Diabetes itself does not lead to early death. It is because diabetes causes so many other problems (e.g. with the heart and kidneys) that those with diabetes can have a shorter lifespan. That is why it is important for health professionals to identify and help manage diabetes early. Doing so treats other conditions associated with the disease, and reduces the risk of subsequent problems.

This is why a 'multi-team' approach is normally recommended.

IMPACT OF MOUTH ON DIABETES

Inflammation in the mouth increases the risk of getting type-2 diabetes, or makes it harder to control your blood sugar if you already have type 1 or type 2 diabetes. This is because inflammation can have a direct impact on the pancreas, the organ in the body where insulin is made. Inflammation can also have an indirect effect on insulin resistance and control of sugar levels.[12]

There is also an enzyme (enzymes are produced by the body to help turn things we eat and drink into products that the body can use) called salivatan. This enzyme is believed to stimulate insulin release, so having a dry mouth will have a direct impact on diabetes.[13]

Inflammation in the mouth can impact on diabetes in the three pathways seen in Image 9.

1. Mouth inflammation triggers the pro-inflammatory state. Certain mediators can affect the beta cells in the pancreas, having an impact on risk of diabetes and glycaemic control (the red arrows).

2. Some of these mediators can have an effect on the way our cells respond to insulin, creating so-called insulin resistance. This will have an impact on the risk of someone getting diabetes and also on glycaemic control (the blue arrows).

3. These mediators can affect the liver and increase the release of further mediators (such as CRP). These can also have an effect on insulin resistance (the green arrows).

Smoking will impact on both the risk of developing diabetes, and the likelihood of complications in those who have diabetes. It will increase the risk of type 2 diabetes directly.

---

12 Donahue, R. P. and Wu, T., 'Insulin Resistance and Periodontal Disease: An Epidemiologic Overview of Research Needs and Future Directions', *Ann. Periodontol.* 6/1 (2001), 119–24.

13 Kimua, I. et al., 'Reduction of Incretin-like Salivatin in Saliva from Patients with Type 2 Diabetes and in Parotid Glands of Stretozotocin-diabetic BALB/c Mice', *Diabs. Obes. Metab.* 3/4 (2001), 254–8.

If you smoke and you already have diabetes, you are at an increased risk of developing complications when compared to non-smokers with diabetes.

IMPACT OF DIABETES ON THE MOUTH

Those with diabetes are at an increased risk of dry mouth, decay, oral thrush, and gum disease which all, in turn, lead to oral inflammation.[14] They are twice as likely to have gum disease as those

---

14 Fernandes, J. K. et al., 'Periodontal Disease Status in Gullah African Americans with Type 2 Diabetes Living in South Carolina', *J. Periodontol.*, 80/7 (2009), 1062–8.

Mealy, B L. and Ocampo, G. L., 'Diabetes Mellitus and Periodontal Disease', *Periodontol.2000*, 44/1 (2007), 127–53.

Campus, G. et al., 'Diabetes and Periodontal Disease: A Case-Control Study', *J. Periodontol.*, 6/3 (2005), 418–25.

Motegi, K., Nakano, Y., and Ueno, T., 'Clinical Studies on Diabetes Mellitus and Diseases of the Oral Region', *Bulletin of Tokyo Medical & Dental University*, 22/3 (1975), 243–7.

Taylor, G. W., Manz, M. C., and Borgnakke, W. S., 'Diabetes, Periodontal Diseases, Dental Caries and Tooth Loss: A Review of the Literature', *Compendium of Continuing Education in Dentistry*, 25/3 (2004), 179–90.

Soskolne, A., 'The Relationship Between Periodontal Disease and Diabetes: An Overview', Ann. *Periodontol.*, 6/1 (2001), 91–8.

Mealy, B. L., 'Periodontal Disease and Diabetes: A Two Way Street', *J. Am. Dent. Assoc.*, 137/suppl. (2006), 26s–31s.

Taylor, G. W. et al., 'Severe Periodontitis and Risk for Poor Glycemic Control in Patients with Non-Insulin Dependent Diabetes Mellitus', *J. Periodontol.*, 67/suppl. 10 (1996), 1085–93.

Grossi, S. G., 'Treatment of Periodontal Disease and Control of Diabetes: An Assessment of the Evidence and Need for Future Research', *Ann. Periodontol.*, 6/1 (2001), 138–145.

Moore, P. A. et al., 'Type 1 Diabetes Mellitus, Xerostomia, and Salivary Flow Rates', *Oral Surg., Oral Med., Oral Path., Radiol., Endod.*, 92/3 (2001), 281–91.

Sreebny, L. M. et al., 'Xerostomia in Diabetes Mellitus', *Diabetes Care*, 15/7 (1992), 900–4.

Zegarelli, D J., 'Fungal Infections of the Oral Cavity', Otolaryngol. *Clin. North Am.*, 23/6 (1993), 1069–89.

Thorstensson, H. and Hugoson, A., 'Periodontal Disease Experience in Adult Long-Duration Insulin-Dependant Diabetics', *J. Clin. Periodontol.*, 20/5 (1993), 352–8.

Taylor, G. W. et al., 'Non-insulin Dependent Diabetes Mellitus and Alveolar Bone Loss Progression Over Two Years', *J. Periodontol.*, 69/1 (1998), 76–83.

without diabetes. Any worsening of gum disease in someone with diabetes can be an indicator that kidney failure may follow.[15]

We all produce a fluid in the gums called gingival crevicular fluid. If blood-sugar levels are higher than is ideal, some of this sugar will be released with the gingival crevicular fluid 'feeding' the bacteria that cause gum disease.

If you have diabetes, you are more likely to get decay if your blood sugars are high. I mentioned gingival crevicular fluid earlier. When blood-sugar levels are higher than is ideal, some of this sugar will be released with the gingival crevicular fluid. Once again this 'feeds' the bacteria that cause decay.

DIABETES VICIOUS CIRCLE

So this is the real crux of diabetes and oral health management. We have seen that diabetes can have a devastating impact on oral health, and that oral health can have an impact on diabetes. This creates a vicious circle.

A patient with periodontal (gum) disease and diabetes is eight times more likely to die a premature death than someone with diabetes who has healthy, well-managed gums.[16]

Not only is gum disease more common in those with diabetes, but we see more severe gum disease, which is also harder to treat. The

---

15 Mealy, B. L., 'Periodontal Disease and Diabetes: A Two Way Street', *J. Am. Dent. Assoc.*, 137/ suppl. (2006), 26s–31s.

Shultis, W. A. et al., 'Effect of Periodontitis on Overt Nephropathy and End-Stage Renal Disease in Type 2 Diabetes', *Diabetes Care*, 30/2 (2007), 306–11.

16 Saremi, A. et al., 'Periodontal Disease and Mortality in Type 2 Diabetes', *Diabetes Care*, 28/1 (2005), 27–32.

statistics show two to three times the occurrence of gum disease in those with diabetes.[17]

PRE-DIABETES

This is a condition worth identifying at this point. Someone with pre-diabetes (also called impaired glucose regulation/impaired fasting glucose/impaired glucose tolerance) has five to fifteen times the risk of developing diabetes when compared to others.[18] Progression to diabetes is not inevitable, and there are interventions (both from the oral health aspect and other changes such as diet, exercise, and smoking cessation) which will reduce the risk of the progression to type 2 diabetes.[19]

TOOLS THAT THE DENTIST CAN USE

The 'diabetes-dental matrix' is a tool that I have developed. It is a computer-based measuring system that enables us to

17   Mealy, B L. and Ocampo, G. L., 'Diabetes Mellitus and Periodontal Disease', *Periodontol.2000*, 44/1 (2007), 127–53.

Grant-Theule, D., 'Periodontal Disease, Diabetes and Immune Response: A Review of Current Concepts', *J. West. Soc. Periodontol. Periodontal Abs.*, 44/3 (1996), 69–77.

Loe, H. and Genco, R. J., 'Oral Complications in Diabetes', <http://www.diabetes.niddk.nih.gov/dm/pubs/america/pdf/chapter23.pdf>.

Lamster, I. B. et al., 'The Relationship between Oral Health and Diabetes Mellitus', *JADA*, 139 (suppl., 2008), 19s–24s.

Taylor, G. W. and Borgnakke, W. S., 'Periodontal Disease: Associations with Diabetes, Glycaemic Control, and Complications', *Oral Dis.*, 14/3 (2008), 191–203.

18   Santaguida, P. L. et al., 'Diagnosis, Prognosis, and Treatment of Impaired Glucose Tolerance and Impaired Fasting Glucose', *Evid. Rep. Technol. Assess.*, 128 (Summer 2005), 1–11.

19   Diabetes UK, Prediabetes: Preventing the Type 2 Diabetes Epidemic, report, <http://www.diabetes.org.uk/Documents/Reports/PrediabetesPreventingtheType2diabetesepidemicOct2009report.pdf>.

assess the aspects of the mouth that influence diabetes, and the aspects of diabetes that influence the mouth. This means we can see how one impacts on the other, and offer solutions to help improve both. Dentists affiliated with the Diabetes and Dentistry Organisation use this tool to help them choose the most appropriate care for patients.

My own published work on the matrix showed how it can be used by dentists and their teams to identify the areas of the mouth that are most likely having an impact on diabetes control, so that we can intervene where most appropriate.[20]

A version of the matrix can be used for those at risk of getting any of the diseases discussed in this book and addressing the areas of inflammation will help prevent the risk of developing the disease.

SCREENING FOR DIABETES IN DENTAL PRACTICE

It is estimated that 850,000 people in the UK have undiagnosed diabetes. If they wait until they get symptoms, they are very likely to have irreversible organ damage. Statistically, more than half a million of these people regularly visit their dentist. By carrying out screening in dental practices, we can help identify those with diabetes so they can be treated before irreversible organ damage occurs. We can also identify many more who are at risk so they can hopefully take measures to avoid getting diabetes. I am a supporter of screening

20 Guyver, R. P., 'Diabetes and Dental Interface: A Measuring and Management Tool for Primary-Care Dental Practitioners and their Teams', *Minerva Endocrinologica*, 37, suppl. 1 (2012), 106.

Guyver, R. P., 'Diabetes and Dental Interface: A Measuring and Management Tool for Primary-Care Dental Practitioners and their Teams', *Diabetes Care*, (Fall 2012 suppl.), 21.

in the dental setting. This screening can take the form of a simple questionnaire to identify those at risk (who are then asked to see their doctor). Dentists who are prepared to do more for their patients can include a simple finger-prick test to see if blood sugar levels are within normal limits. I do this for my patients. If you are a dentist who is interested in how you can introduce diabetes screening to help your patients out, please email me at expert@diabetesanddentistry. co.uk, and I'll be glad to help you set up a screening programme.

After just one year of introducing this at my practice, I identified a number of patients with undiagnosed diabetes, and many more who are at risk and so can do things to reduce their risk of developing type 2 diabetes later on.

JANET'S STORY (BASED ON A PRESS RELEASE)

Name has been changed to protect identity

Sixty-five-year-old Janet Dawson had every reason to believe that she was in good health for her age.

'I didn't go to the gym but I made sure I did plenty of walking', says the retired building-society cashier.

'I knew I was overweight. I was only five foot four and weighed nearly twelve and a half stone, but I always had plenty of energy and rarely felt ill.'

In fact, Janet was already in the early stages of type 2 diabetes.

But without any discernible symptoms, Janet would undoubtedly have gone undiagnosed for many more months, if not years (by which time her condition would have already begun to cause irreparable damage to her body).

As Janet had some of the risk factors, when she visited us for a Healthy Mouth Review (see the section 'What can my dental team do?') in July 2012, she was offered diabetes screening, a system we devised from Diabetes UK recommendations. In Janet's words:

"I filled in a questionnaire and Richard did a finger-prick blood test. My blood sugar was extremely high and Richard said that this could mean that I had type 2 diabetes and asked me to come back for a glucose fasting test the following morning. This test confirmed I had high blood sugar. Later that week my GP carried out blood tests and I was diagnosed with the condition. I was really shocked. I had absolutely none of the symptoms that you usually associate with diabetes. I wasn't thirsty and wasn't constantly going to the loo. However, thanks to Richard, I had been diagnosed at a very early stage before any damage was done. I didn't need medication and was told that if I lost weight I may even reverse the diagnosis."

Janet has already lost one and half stone and her blood sugar has dropped from 8.5 to 6. She is also paying careful attention to her oral health.

"I feel I have been extremely lucky to be diagnosed so early and I want to make the most of that chance. The last thing I want is to be put on medication. My GP asked how I came to him when I didn't have symptoms. When I told him my

dentist had picked it up, he was very impressed. I think all
dentists should be carrying out this basic test."

ROLE OF DENTAL MEDICINE IN DIABETES

There is plenty of evidence that dentists can have a positive impact by helping to reduce the risk of someone getting type 2 diabetes, and a positive impact on diabetes control-for both types 1 and 2. Ensuring good oral health (by eliminating inflammation) will put you in a position where the risk of getting this disease and all its side effects can be minimised. If you already suffer from the disease, removal of oral inflammation will help your blood-sugar control. Good diabetes control improves oral health. This is one of the diseases in which the vicious circle exists.

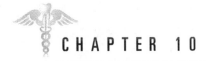

CHAPTER 10

Atheromatous (Arterial) Disease

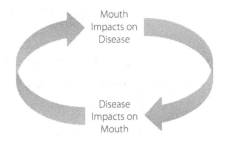

Mouth Impacts on Disease

Disease Impacts on Mouth

What is atheromatous (arterial) disease? Atheromatous disease occurs when so-called plaques develop in the blood vessels (in particular the arteries). It is a very common disease and contributes to about one-third of all deaths in the UK each year through strokes, heart attacks, and clots in the lungs. It has a significant effect on peoples' health, and in 2004 a study showed that sixty-nine million workdays in the U.K. were lost as a result of heart disease alone, and the cost to the NHS of managing heart disease and strokes, not including lost work days, is in excess of £20 billion per year.[21]

---

21 BBC News, (May 2006) <http:// news.bbc.co.uk/1/hi/health/4764891.stm>.

National Audit Office, (Nov 2005) <http://www.nao.org.uk/whats_new/0506/0506452.aspx>.

Atheromatous disease is actually a group of diseases. Image 10 shows one way to look at the different parts of the body that are affected.

When plaques cause a blockage, the part of the body supplied by the affected blood vessels is starved of oxygen, resulting in damage to that part of the body. Sometimes pieces of the plaque break away or rupture, which also causes damage.

Often, health concerns such as a heart attack, stroke, and so on, are examples that the damage has occurred.

IMPACT OF MOUTH ON ATHEROMATOUS (ARTERIAL) DISEASE

There is a link between mouth inflammation and both the formation and rupture of these harmful plaques.[22] C-reactive protein (CRP) is one of the factors that increase the risk of atheromatous disease. We saw earlier that mouth inflammation will cause CRP to be released in the body. Chronic inflammation also underlies the process of plaque formation. Studies over the last twenty years have shown links between mouth inflammation (in particular from gum disease) and atheromatous disease. The severity of gum disease has been shown to be linked to increasing risk of atheromatous disease

---

22 Scannapieco, F. A., Bush, R. B., and Paju, S., 'Associations between Periodontal Disease and Risk for Atherosclerosis, Cardiovascular Disease, and Stroke: A Systematic Review', *Ann. Periodontol.*, 8/1 (2003), 38–53.

Meurman, J. H., Sanz, M., and Janket, S. J., 'Oral Health, Atherosclerosis and Cardiovascular Disease', *Crit. Rev. Oral Biol. Med.*, 15/6 (2004), 403–13.

Khader, Y. S., Albashaireh, Z. S., and Alomari, M. A., 'Periodontal Diseases and the Risk of Coronary Heart and Cerebrovascular Diseases: A Meta-analysis', *J. Periodontol.*, 75/8 (2004), 1046–53.

Vettore, M. V., 'Periodontal Disease and Cardiovascular Disease', *Evid. Based Dent.*, 5 (2004), 69.

and its consequences.[23] There are numerous other studies that have established links between the two.

There are also studies which show that by treating oral inflammation, the 'serum markers' (i.e. things that your doctor detects in blood tests) for atheromatous disease were reduced.[24]

It has been shown that mouth inflammation is associated with increased cholesterol levels.[25] It has also been shown that after this inflammation is reduced, cholesterol levels can be decreased.[26]

Let's look at some of the conditions that come under the heading of atheromatous (arterial) disease.

HIGH BLOOD PRESSURE (HYPERTENSION)

About one-third of adults in the UK have hypertension. This increases the risk of having kidney failure, a heart attack, or a stroke.

There is a clear association between CRP and high blood pressure.[27]

23 Beck, J. D. et al., 'Periodontal Disease and Cardiovascular Disease', *J. Periodontol.*, 67/10 Sppl. (1996), 1123–37.

Wu, T. et al., 'An Examination of the Relation between Periodontal Health Status and Cardiovascular Risk Factors: Serum Total and HDL Cholesterol, C- Reactive Protein, and Plasma Fibrinogen', *Am. J. Epidemiol.*, 151/3 (2000), 273-82.

DeStefano, F. et al., 'Dental Disease and the Risk of Coronary Heart Disease and Mortality', *Br. Med. J.*, 306/6879 (1993), 688–91.

24 Joshipura, K. J. et al., 'Periodontal Disease and Biomarkers Related to Cardiovascular Disease', *J. Dent. Res.*, 83/2 (2004), 151–5.

25 Iacaponio, A. M. and Cutler, C. W., 'Pathophysiological Relationship between Periodontitis and Systemic Disease: Recent Concepts Involving Serum Lipids', *J. Periodontol.*, 71/8 (2000), 1375–84.

Katz, J. et al., 'Association between Periodontal Pockets and Elevated Cholesterol and Low density Lipoprotein Cholesterol Levels', *J. Periodontol.*, 73/5 (2002), 494–500.

26 D'Aiuto, F. et al., 'Short-Term Effects of Intensive Periodontal Therapy on Serum Inflammatory Markers and Cholesterol', J. Dent. Res., 84/3 (2005), 269–73.

27 Sesso, H. D. et al., 'C-reactive Protein and the Risk of Developing Hypertension', *JAMA*, 290/22 (2003), 2945–51.

HEART ATTACK (MYOCARDIAL INFARCTION) AND
STROKE (CEREBROVASCULAR ACCIDENT)

QUICK FACTS: STROKES AND HEART ATTACKS

People often mistakenly use these terms, thinking they are the same. A heart attack occurs when a piece of muscle of the heart dies because it has been starved of oxygen. A stroke occurs when a section of the brain is damaged because it has been starved of oxygen.

Heart attack is the major cause of death from heart disease. There are around 100,000 people who suffer heart attacks in the UK each year. One in three people who have a heart attack die before they get to hospital.

The existence of periodontal disease has been shown as a predictor for a heart attack. One study showed that people with gum disease or an infection in a tooth were 30% more likely to have a heart attack than individuals who did not have these oral infections.[28] It has also been shown that heart attack risk increases with the severity of gum disease.[29]

---

28 Matilla, K. et al., 'Association between Dental Health and Acute Myocardial Infarction', *Br. Med. J.*, 298/6676 (1989), 779–82.

29 Beck, J. D. et al., 'Periodontal Disease and Cardiovascular Disease', *J. Periodontol.*, 67/10 Sppl. (1996), 1123–37.

Wu, T. et al., 'An Examination of the Relation between Periodontal Health Status and Cardiovascular Risk Factors: Serum Total and HDL Cholesterol, C- Reactive Protein, and Plasma Fibrinogen', *Am. J. Epidemiol.*, 151/3 (2000), 273-82.

DeStefano, F. et al., 'Dental Disease and the Risk of Coronary Heart Disease and Mortality', *Br. Med. J.*, 306/6879 (1993), 688–91.

Other studies show that there is a link between mouth inflammation and stroke.[30]

High levels of CRP are a strong predictor of future heart attack and stroke and we have already seen that mouth inflammation increases CRP levels.[31]

HEART SURGERY

The implications of an infection from the mouth following heart surgery are so significant that I am often asked to assess patients prior to surgery. I am checking for, and treating, any areas of infection or inflammation. This is because of the high risk that bacteria from the mouth will significantly damage the heart following surgery.

PERIPHERAL VASCULAR DISEASE

This disease results in reduced blood supply, particularly to the legs and feet. It can cause no symptoms initially, developing gradually to pain on walking and eventually pain at rest. The pain occurs as the muscles are starved of the oxygen they need. Ultimately it can result in gangrene and the need for amputation.

There do not appear to be any quality studies looking at the links between oral health and peripheral vascular disease. However, it

30 Joshipura, K. J. et al., 'Periodontal Disease, Tooth Loss, and Incidence of Ischaemic Stroke', *Stroke.*, 34/1 (2003), 47–52.

Grau, A. J. et al., 'Association between Acute Cerebrovascular Ischaemia and Chronic and Recurrent Infection', *Stroke.*, 28/9 (1997), 1724–29.

Elter, J. et al., 'Relationship of Periodontal Disease and Edentulism to Stroke/TIA', *J. Dent. Res.*, 82/12 (2003), 998–1001.

31 Ridker, P. M. et al., 'Inflammation, Aspirin, and the Risk of Cardiovascular Disease in Apparently Healthy Men', *N. Engl. J. Med.*, 336/14 (1997), 973–9.

is reasonable to believe that a link may be found in the future, given that the disease process is similar to that of atherosclerosis.

ROLE OF DENTAL MEDICINE IN ATHEROMATOUS (ARTERIAL) DISEASE

This is another disease, which we can help avoid by ensuring that there is no oral inflammation. We can also reduce its impact if it already exists. Dental Medicine Experts will be aware of the impact of oral health on atheromatous (arterial) disease, and of the significant positive impact we can have on our patients' health and lifespan. Here again, a vicious circle exists.

CHAPTER 11

Lung Disease

Due to the close proximity of the mouth to the airways, it stands to reason that oral health could have an impact on the lungs. After all, when you breathe through your mouth, the air goes straight into your lungs. Just as the wind can blow a piece of grit or dust into your eye, breathing can carry bugs from the mouth into the lungs. Recent research confirms links, particularly links between levels of plaque and gum disease with pneumonia and chronic obstructive pulmonary disease (COPD). These could be direct links, particularly as most adults inhale small amounts of the fluid from the mouth when breathing through their mouths, especially when asleep. If there is gum disease or increased levels of plaque, there will be increased levels of bacteria. Inhaling these bacteria can cause problems in the lungs. Alternatively the link may be related to the process of inflammation, as we have seen in the case of diabetes and atheromatous disease. It may even be true that both pathways exist. This is an area of ongoing research.

COPD

What is COPD? Chronic obstructive pulmonary disease (COPD) is the term used to describe three conditions: chronic asthma, chronic bronchitis, and emphysema. It affects about three million people in the UK, although it is believed about two million of these are not diagnosed.[32] Thirty thousand deaths per year are attributable to COPD.[33] Smoking is the main cause of COPD, although like all diseases, other factors play a role. Remember earlier when we looked at multifactorial disease? Chronic bronchitis is a common condition affecting approximately a quarter of the population over the age of forty-five.

Acute flare-ups of COPD cause periods of more severe symptoms often associated with bacterial infections.

IMPACT OF MOUTH ON COPD

Studies have shown links between oral health and increased risk of COPD, even when taking other risk factors into consideration.[34] In one study the risk of an acute flare-up was also directly related to decayed teeth.[35] Increased loss of bone through gum disease has been directly related to a reduction in lung function.[36]

---

32 National Institute for Health and Clinical Excellence, Chronic Obstructive Pulmonary Disease Costing Report, <http://www.nice.org.uk/nicemedia/live/13029/53292/53292.pdf>.

33 Hicks, Rob, 'Chronic Obstructive Pulmonary Disease (COPD)', BBC,<http://www.bbc.co.uk/health/physical_health/conditions/copd1.shtml>.

34 Scannapieco, F. A., Papadonatos, G. D., and Dunford, R. G., 'Associations between Oral Conditions and Respiratory Disease in a National Sample Survey Population', *Ann. Periodontol.*, 3/1 (1998), 251–6.

Hayes, C. et al., 'The Association between Alveolar Bone Loss and Pulmonary Function: The VA Dental Longitudinal Study', *Ann. Periodontol.*, 3/1 (1998), 257-61.

Scannapieco, F. A. and Ho, A. W., 'Potential Associations between Chronic Respiratory Disease and Periodontal Disease: Analysis of National Health and Nutrition Examination Survey III', *J. Periodontol.*, 72/1 (2001), 50–6.

35 Scannapieco, F. A., Papadonatos, G. D., and Dunford, R. G., 'Associations between Oral Conditions and Respiratory Disease in a National Sample Survey Population', *Ann. Periodontol.*, 3/1 (1998), 251–6.

36 Scannapieco, F. A. and Ho, A. W., 'Potential Associations between Chronic Respiratory Disease and Periodontal Disease: Analysis of National Health and Nutrition Examination Survey III', *J. Periodontol.*, 72/1 (2001), 50–6.

As previously noted the mechanism of action is most likely a direct effect of inhaling bacteria/plaque from the mouth which then goes into an already compromised lung. This is an area of research that is ongoing, but it reinforces the benefits of good oral health on general health.

PNEUMONIA

What is pneumonia? Pneumonia occurs when the lungs get infected. It leads to the inability for oxygen to get from the lungs into the blood stream. It accounts for about 5% of deaths in the UK.

IMPACT OF MOUTH ON PNEUMONIA

Research shows that a visit to the dentist reduces the risk of community acquired pneumonia (CAP).[37] Other studies have shown similar associations.[38] Many of the bacteria which cause CAP are found in the mouth. Some studies show that the use of antibacterial agents in the mouth can reduce the risk of pneumonia in patients in intensive care units (ICUs) in hospitals.[39] Other studies show a

---

37 Almirall, J. et al., 'New Evidence of Risk Factors for Community Acquired Pneumonia: A Population-Based Study: Community Acquired Pneumonia in Catalan Countries, Study Group', *Eur. Respir. J.,* 31/6 (2008), 1274–84.

38 Scannapieco, F. A., Bush, R. B., and Paju, S., 'Associations between Periodontal Disease and Risk for Atherosclerosis, Cardiovascular Disease, and Stroke: A Systematic Review', *Ann. Periodontol.,* 8/1 (2003), 38–53.

Azarpazhooh, A. and Leake, J. L., 'Systematic Review of the Association between Respiratory Diseases and Oral Health', *J. Periodontol.,* 77/9 (2006), 1465–82.

Chan, E. Y. et al., 'Oral Decontamination for Prevention of Pneumonia in Mechanically Ventilated Adults: Systematic Review and Meta-analysis', *BMJ,* 334 (2007), 889.

39 Scannapieco, F. A., Bush, R. B., and Paju, S., 'Associations between Periodontal Disease and Risk for Atherosclerosis, Cardiovascular Disease, and Stroke: A Systematic Review', *Ann. Periodontol.,* 8/1 (2003), 38–53.

reduced risk of CAP in patients who use daily antibacterial mouth-washes in addition to tooth-brushing.[40] This reinforces the likely link.

ROLE OF DENTAL MEDICINE IN LUNG DISEASE

Again, there is plenty of evidence that by ensuring good oral health, we can have a positive impact on the risk of developing certain lung diseases and even reduce the risk of worsening lung diseases if they already exist. Given how common lung disease is, and the role the mouth plays, Dental Medicine Experts help ensure their patients' mouths are not likely to worsen or trigger lung problems.

Azarpazhooh, A. and Leake, J. L., 'Systematic Review of the Association between Respiratory Diseases and Oral Health', J. Periodontol., 77/9 (2006), 1465–82.

Chan, E. Y. et al., 'Oral Decontamination for Prevention of Pneumonia in Mechanically Ventilated Adults: Systematic Review and Meta-analysis', BMJ, 334 (2007), 889.

40 Yoshida, M. et al., 'Oral Care and Pneumonia', Lancet, 354/9177 (1999), 515.

Yoneyama, T. et al., 'Oral Care Reduces Pneumonia in Patients in Nursing Homes', J. Am. Geriatr. Soc., 50/3 (2002), 430–3.

CHAPTER 12

Pregnancy Complications

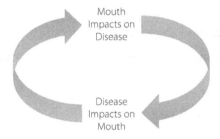

What are pregnancy complications? This term refers to a number of conditions, also known as adverse pregnancy outcomes. They are all significant as they can impact on the health of the baby and/or the mother. Complications include pre-eclampsia (high blood pressure due to pregnancy), pre-term or premature birth, low-birth-weight babies, and miscarriage.

IMPACT OF THE MOUTH ON PREGNANCY COMPLICATIONS

The first evidence linking periodontal disease to pregnancy complications emerged seventeen years ago.[41] Since then, many studies have strengthened the connection. Inflammation in the mouth can

---

41 Offenbacher, S. et al., 'Periodontal Infection as a Possible Risk Factor for Preterm Low Birth Weight', *J. Periodontol.*, 67/10 suppl. (1996), 1103–13.

increase the risk of premature birth, low-birth-weight babies, miscarriage, and pre-eclampsia.[42] There is also evidence that the bacteria that cause gum inflammation can cause amniotic fluid inflammation in mothers who deliver early, possibly affecting the health of their babies.[43] One study showed that untreated gum disease increased the risk of having a pre-term baby fivefold.[44] The risk of having any 'adverse pregnancy outcome' is 7.5 times higher in those with periodontal disease when compared to those who are free of periodontal disease.[45]

Other studies have shown that by intervening and helping reduce inflammation in the mouth, the risk of these adverse outcomes is reduced.[46]

42   Vergnes, J. N. and Sixou, M., 'Preterm Low Birth Weight and Maternal Periodontal Status: A Meta-analysis', *Am. J. Obstet. Gynecol.,* 196/2 (2007), 135.e1–7.

Boggess, K. A. et al., 'Maternal Periodontal Disease Is Associated with an Increased Risk of Pre-eclampsia', *Obstet. Gynecol.,* 101/2 (2003), 227–31.

43   Berfield, C. et al., 'Possible Association between Amniotic Fluid Micro-Organism Infection and Microflora in the Mouth', *BJOG,* 109/5 (2002), 527–33.

44   Lopez, N. J. et al., 'Periodontal Therapy Reduces the Rate of Preterm Low Birth Weight in Women with Pregnancy-Associated Gingivitis', *J. Periodontol.,* 76/ 11suppl. (2005), 2144–53.

45   Bobetis, Y. A., Baros, S. P., and Offenbacher, S., 'Exploring the Relationship between Periodontal Disease and Adverse Pregnancy Outcomes: A Systematic Review', *Br. J. Obst. Gynecol.,* 137 (2006), 135–143.

46   Lopez, N. J. et al., 'Periodontal Therapy Reduces the Rate of Preterm Low Birth Weight in Women with Pregnancy-Associated Gingivitis', *J. Periodontol.,* 76/ 11suppl. (2005), 2144–53.

Lopez, N. J., Smith, P. C., and Gutierrez, J., 'Periodontal Therapy May Reduce the Risk of Pre-term Low Birth Weight in Women with Periodontal Disease: A Randomised Control Trial', *J. Periodontol.,* 73/8 (2002), 911–24.

Jeffcoat, M. K. et al., 'Periodontal Disease and Pre-term Birth: Results of a Pilot Intervention Study', *J. Periodontol.,* 74/8 (2003), 1214–18.

Terannum, F. and Faizuddin, M., 'Effect of Periodontal Therapy on Pregnancy Outcome in Women Affected by Periodontitis', *J. Periodontol.,* 78/11 (2007), 2095–2103.

IMPACT OF PREGNANCY ON THE MOUTH

Pregnancy also has a direct effect on the health of gums, and can worsen existing gum inflammation. It is another example of a vicious circle which Dental Medicine Experts aim to manage.[47]

ROLE OF DENTAL MEDICINE IN PREGNANCY

Due to the links that have been scientifically established, it is prudent to make sure your gums are healthy before you become pregnant.

Approximately three out of four pregnant women have gum inflammation.[48] If you are already pregnant, do not put off a visit to the dentist. It is important that you do all you can to ensure your mouth is as healthy as possible. Ideally, choose a dentist who subscribes to the philosophy of Dental Medicine.

---

47 Offenbacher, S. et al., 'Periodontal Infection as a Possible Risk Factor for Preterm Low Birth Weight', *J. Periodontol.*, 67/10 suppl. (1996), 1103–13.

48 Offenbacher, S. et al., 'Periodontal Infection as a Possible Risk Factor for Preterm Low Birth Weight', *J. Periodontol.*, 67/10 suppl. (1996), 1103–13.

CHAPTER 13

Erectile Dysfunction/ Impotence

S orry guys, you didn't think that you were going to get away with it did you? It has been shown that men in their thirties with inflamed gums are three times more likely to suffer from erectile dysfunction. The process is thought to be linked to the impact that gum inflammation has on vascular diseases. It has also been shown that there was a higher incidence of decay and missing teeth in men with erectile dysfunction compared to men who did not have the condition.[49]

ROLE OF DENTAL MEDICINE ON ERECTILE DYSFUNCTION

This research is relatively new. However, if there is a link between gum inflammation and erectile dysfunction, it further reinforces the philosophy behind Dental Medicine and the interplay between the mouth and general health.

---

49 Oguz, F. et al., 'Is There a Relationship between Chronic Periodontitis and Erectile Dysfunction?', *J. Sex. Med.*, 10/3 (Mar 2013)., 838-43

CHAPTER 14

Dementia and Alzheimer's Disease

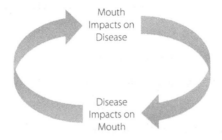

Mouth Impacts on Disease

Disease Impacts on Mouth

What are dementia and Alzheimer's disease? Dementia is a set of symptoms that includes memory loss and problems with communication and reasoning and it can also cause mood changes. Dementia is a progressive disease, which means that the symptoms will gradually worsen. Dementia affects about 820,000 people in the UK, and surprisingly, some of those are under the age of sixty-five. There are several causes, including Alzheimer's disease and vascular dementia (caused by arterial disease). Alzheimer's disease is the most common cause of dementia. It occurs when brain cells die faster than they normally would.

Alzheimer's disease and dementia affect life expectancy by as much as ten years if diagnosed before the age of sixty-five. It can also impact quality of life in sufferers as well as their families and carers.

IMPACT OF THE MOUTH ON DEMENTIA AND ALZHEIMER'S DISEASE

We already know that the mouth plays a role in vascular dementia due to its role in atheromatous (arterial) disease.

At present this remains an area of interesting research. There are some studies which show a link between tooth loss and Alzheimer's disease, and links between gum disease and Alzheimer's disease.[50]

A recent study in California showed a link between dementia and the number of times a day that patients brushed their teeth. Researchers studied almost 5500 people over an eighteen-year period. Those who reported brushing less than once a day were 65% more likely to develop dementia than those who brushed twice a day.[51]

Another study has shown that chewing ability may be related to dementia. Those who struggled to eat hard foods were at an increased risk of dementia. One explanation is that those who struggle to eat hard foods will choose not to, and the reduced amount of chewing reduces blood flow to the brain.[52] So if you find eating hard and

---

50   Gatz, M. et al., 'Potentially Modifiable Risk Factors for Dementia in Identical Twins', *Alzheimer's Dement.,* 2/2 (2006), 110–17.

Shimazaki, Y. et al., 'Influence of Dentition Status on Physical Disability, Mental Impairment, and Mortality in Institutionalised Elderly People', *J. Dent. Res.,* 80/1 (2001), 340–5.

Kondo, K., Niino, M., and Shido, K. A., 'Case Control Study of Alzheimer's Disease in Japan: Significance of Lifestyles', *Dementia,* 5/6 (Nov.–Dec.1994), 314–26.

51   Paganini-Hill, A., White, S. C., and Atchison, K. A., 'Dentition, Dental Habits and Dementia: The Leisure World Cohort Study', *J. Am. Ger. Soc.,* 60/8 (2012), 1556-63.

52   Paganini-Hill, A., White, S. C., and Atchison, K. A., 'Dentition, Dental Habits and Dementia: The Leisure World Cohort Study', *J. Am. Ger. Soc.,* 60/8 (2012), 1556-63.

chewy foods difficult, perhaps a visit with the dentist to discuss your options would be helpful.

IMPACT OF DEMENTIA AND ALZHEIMER'S DISEASE ON THE MOUTH

Dentists who care for those with dementia or Alzheimer's disease have observed that the oral health of these patients worsens as cleaning the mouth becomes difficult to do, and as dementia progresses, making it difficult to remember to do. Even with the best will in the world many carers struggle to make a positive impact on maintaining the oral health of the person they care for. Often the dental work that dentists can perform is severely compromised, especially in the later stages, because of the lack of ability to accept treatment.

ROLE OF DENTAL MEDICINE IN ALZHEIMER'S DISEASE AND DEMENTIA

A lot of this research is relatively new. However, it seems that the impact of the mouth, both via blood flow to the brain from chewing and via the inflammation route is probably having an effect.

If you are keen in finding out more about preventing Alzheimer's and dementia there is a really useful book called *100 Simple things you can do to prevent Alzheimer's and age-related memory loss* by Jean Carper, I can thoroughly recommend reading it.[53]

Over the next few years it is likely that research that will establish the relationship between the mouth and dementia. Yet again, we see the existence of another vicious circle.

Lexomboom, D., Trulsson, M., Wardh, I., and Parker, M. G., 'Chewing Ability and Tooth Loss: Associated with Cognitive Impairment in an Elderley Population Study', *J. Am. Geriatr. Soc.*, 60/10 (2012), 1951–6.

53 ISBN: 978-0-09-193951-9

CHAPTER 15

Cancer

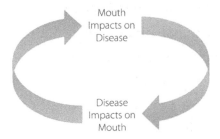

Mouth
Impacts on
Disease

Disease
Impacts on
Mouth

C ancer costs the NHS about £10 billion each year.[54] It directly affects about one in three of us during our lives, and leads to more than 150,000 deaths per year in the UK.[55]

Like the dementia link, this is an active area of research. To examine it, let's look at oral cancer and other cancers separately.

WHAT IS ORAL AND PHARYNGEAL CANCER?

There are nearly 6000 cases of oral cancer diagnosed each year in the UK. More than 1800 people die from it each year. If diagnosed

---

54 BUPA, 'Cost of Cancer,' http://www.bupa.co.uk/intermediaries/int-news/int-bupa-updates/cost-of-cancer-report.

55 NHS, 'Cancer Survival Rates "Threatened by Rising Cost"', Choices, <http://www.nhs.uk/news/2011/12December/Pages/cancer-treatment-cost-may-increase.aspx>.

Cancer Research UK, 'Cancer Mortality Statistics', <http://www.cancerresearchuk.org/cancer-info/cancerstats/mortality/uk-cancer-mortality-statistics>.

early, the survival rate (over five years) is as high as 90%.[56] As with any disease, prevention is better than cure, so if we can help our patients avoid it, what a great service that is to them.

IMPACT OF THE MOUTH ON ORAL AND PHARYNGEAL CANCER

Studies from as far back as thirty-five years ago demonstrated an increased risk of oral cancer in those with gum inflammation, even when factors like smoking and alcohol were taken into account.[57] Other studies have since backed up these findings.[58] Interestingly, it appears that the influence of gum inflammation in females is greater than it is in males, but it is still relevant to both sexes.[59]

Evidence suggests that the risk of oral cancer is influenced by oral hygiene, gum inflammation, and gum disease.

IMPACT OF THE MOUTH ON OTHER FORMS OF CANCER

There are studies showing possible links between oral health and the following cancer types:

---

56 British Dental Health Foundation, Mouth Cancer Action (home page), www.mouthcancer.org.

57 Graham, S. et al., 'Dentition, Diet, Tobacco and Alcohol in the Epidemiology of Oral Cancer', J. Natl. *Cancer Inst.,* 59/6 (1977), 1611–18.

58 Rosenquist, K. et al., 'Oral Status, Oral Infections, and some Lifestyle Factors as Risk Factors for Oral and Oropharyngeal Squamous Cell Carcinoma: A Population-Based Case Control Study in Southern Sweden', *Acta Otolaryngol.,* 125/12 (2005), 1327–36.

Rezende, C. P. et al., 'Oral Health Changes in Patients with Oral and Oropharyngeal Cancer', *Braz. J. Otorhinolaryngol.,* 74/4 (2008), 596–600.

Tezal, M. et al., 'Chronic Periodontitis and the Risk of Tongue Cancer', *Arch. Otolaryngol. Head Neck Surg.,* 133/5 (2007), 450–4.

59 Zheng, T. Z. et al., 'Dentition, Oral Hygiene, and Risk of Oral Cancer: A Case Control Study in Beijing, People's Republic of China', *Cancer Causes & Control,* 1/3 (1990), 235–41.

- gastric and oesophageal cancers[60]
- colon/bowel cancer[61]
- lung cancer[62]
- pancreatic cancer[63]
- kidney cancer[64]
- haematological cancer (e.g. leukaemia, lymphoma, myeloma)[65]

There is a lot of work for the medical and dental academics to do in these areas. However, enough evidence is already there for us to take note and want to ensure we are doing all we can to optimise oral health. Some of the links between oral health and cancer may be due to a direct relationship, for example, gastric, oesophageal, and lung cancer. Remember that I mentioned bacteria are carried into

---

60 Abnet, C. C. et al., 'Prospective Study of Tooth Loss and Incident Eosophageal and Gastric Cancers in China', *Cancer Causes & Control,* 12/9 (2001), 847–54.

Watabe, K. et al., 'Lifestyle and Gastric Cancer: A Case-Control Study', *Oncol. Rep.,* 5/5 (1998), 1191–94.

61 Dentistry, 'Possible Link between Gum Disease and Bowel Cancer', 13 Feb. 2012, <http://www.dentistry.co.uk/news/possible-link-between-gum-disease-and-bowel-cancer>.

62 Hujoel, P. P. et al., 'An Exploration of the Periodontitis-Cancer Association', *Ann. Epidemiol.,* 13/5 (2003), 312–16.

Michaud, D. S. et al., 'Periodontal Disease, Tooth Loss, and Cancer Risk in Male Health Professionals: A Prospective Cohort Study', *Lancet Oncol.,* 9/6 (2008), 550–8.

63 Michaud, D. S. et al., 'Periodontal Disease, Tooth Loss, and Cancer Risk in Male Health Professionals: A Prospective Cohort Study', *Lancet Oncol.,* 9/6 (2008), 550–8.

Stolzenberg-Solomon, R. Z. et al., 'Tooth Loss, Pancreatic Cancer, and Helicobacter Pylori', *Am. J. Clin. Nutr.,* 78/1 (2003), 176–81.

Michaud, D. S. et al., 'A Prospective Study of Periodontal Disease and Pancreatic Cancer in US Male Health Professionals', *J. Nat. Cancer Inst.,* 99/2 (2007), 171–5.

64 Michaud, D. S. et al., 'Periodontal Disease, Tooth Loss, and Cancer Risk in Male Health Professionals: A Prospective Cohort Study', *Lancet Oncol.,* 9/6 (2008), 550–8.

65 Michaud, D. S. et al., 'Periodontal Disease, Tooth Loss, and Cancer Risk in Male Health Professionals: A Prospective Cohort Study', *Lancet Oncol.,* 9/6 (2008), 550–8.

the lungs when you breathe? Well, when you eat and drink, bacteria are carried into the stomach. They may also have a direct effect there. Alternatively the link may be explained by inflammation, as we have seen previously for other diseases.

IMPACT OF CANCER ON THE MOUTH

Many cancer drugs can have an impact on the mouth, leading to ulcers, soreness and dry mouth. These side effects mean that people on these drugs are often more likely to have decay and gum disease. So help from their dental team is needed. The team should be prepared to intervene early should anything start to deteriorate.

Radiotherapy to the head and neck has significant effects on the mouth, both in the short and the long term. In the short term it can lead to extreme discomfort and difficulty in swallowing (essentially the patient will have radiation burns in the mouth and throat). In severe cases these need to be dealt with in a hospital setting. When I worked in the maxillofacial surgery unit in the hospital, I cared for patients who were undergoing radiotherapy to the head and neck regions. I witnessed first-hand how debilitating and painful radio-therapy was, but it was essential to try and beat the cancer. They were often having this treatment just a short time after they had been through significant surgery. I'm sure if they could have turned the clocks back, they would have done so to ensure an early diagnosis was made and to reduce their exposure to invasive surgery and radiother-apy. Or better still, the cancer might have been prevented completely by removing potential risk factors.

After completion of radiation treatment, patients can be left with salivary glands that do not function (increasing the risk of decay, mouth inflammation, and the unpleasantness of a dry mouth).

The bone that supports teeth can also be affected. Infected teeth or infections following extractions can cause significant damage to the jawbone. Preventing these infections is so essential that when I was working in the hospital, I was often asked to remove all the teeth considered 'at risk', to reduce the risk of bone infections prior to starting radiotherapy.

DIET AND CANCER, A CRITICAL CONNECTION

The mouth can influence cancer in another way. There is mounting evidence of the role of diet in preventing a range of diseases including cancer. Recent research shows that protection is likely to come from fresh vegetables. Studies show that eating cruciferous vegetables (e.g. choy, watercress, broccoli, sprouts, cauliflower, radish, and cabbage) at least once a week will decrease the risk of oral cancer by 17%. It also reduces the risk of kidney cancer by 32%, oesophageal cancer by 28%, and colorectal and breast cancer by 17%. The challenge that people have if they cannot chew properly is discussed in the chapter on 'Diet Nutrition and Chewing Ability' and has a direct impact on diet choices.

ROLE OF DENTAL MEDICINE IN CANCER

Cancer is a frightening and debilitating disease, and Dental Medicine Experts will agree that we should be doing what we can to eradicate oral inflammation in the interest of reducing the risk of cancer. As I'm sure you have spotted, yet another vicious circle exists here.

Oral and pharyngeal cancers are often first identified by dentists. Later in this book I will introduce you to the Healthy Mouth Review. In that section you will see that all dentists should be carefully examining their patients' mouths and necks to detect anything that indicates a cancer may be developing.

CHAPTER 16

Osteoporosis

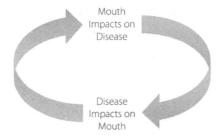

Mouth Impacts on Disease

Disease Impacts on Mouth

What is osteoporosis? In healthy individuals a normal bone remodelling process occurs. It is due to this process that the bone is replaced gradually. You may not be aware that the entire human skeleton is replaced every seven years. It is a dynamic process whereby the bone is resorbed (i.e. eaten up) by osteoclast cells and new bone is made by osteoblast cells. If the balance between these two types of activity is correct, the bone stays strong and healthy. If the osteoclast cell activity is greater than the osteoblast cells, the bone will begin to disappear gradually. It is because of this imbalance that osteoporosis occurs.

Osteoporosis will affect quality of life significantly, and the risk of fracture (particularly of the hip bone) is always of concern. Hip fractures can be severely life limiting and lead to a shortened lifespan.

IMPACT OF THE MOUTH ON OSTEOPOROSIS

Through the process of inflammation, certain messengers called cytokines are released. Cytokines will influence the way osteoclasts and osteoblasts function. Because of this, inflammation in the mouth may have an influence on osteoporosis.

IMPACT OF OSTEOPOROSIS ON THE MOUTH

It is also possible that osteoporosis may accelerate bone loss from around the teeth where there is existing gum disease. Osteoporosis has also been linked to tooth loss.[66]

DENTAL IMPLANTS

Implants are normally the treatment of choice when replacing missing teeth. The presence of osteoporosis needs to be considered, since both osteoporosis and some medications used to treat it can affect the way a dentist plans the implant treatment.

If you are being treated for osteoporosis with one of the group of medications called bisphosphonates, your dentist will need to consider this if you require a tooth extraction or an implant. These medications can affect the bone in such a way that severe infections can develop if appropriate steps are not taken.

---

66   Kaye, E. K., 'Bone Health and Oral Health', *J. Am. Dent. Assoc.,* 138/5 (2007), 616–19.

Lerner, U. H., 'Inflammation-Induced Bone Remodelling in Periodontal Disease and the Role of Post Menopausal Osteoporosis', *J. Dent. Res.,* 85/7 (2006), 596–607.

ROLE OF DENTAL MEDICINE IN OSTEOPOROSIS

Osteoporosis affects many people and can lead to significant problems especially if it causes bone fractures. Dental Medicine Experts will be aiming to reduce the impact of osteoporosis on the mouth, and to reduce the inflammation in the mouth so that it cannot have an effect on osteoporosis.

Teeth are supported by bone; implants are supported by bone. Dental Medicine Experts have knowledge of bone disease and normal bone healing processes as this influences optimal treatment options.

This means osteoporosis is another medical condition where there is a vicious circle.

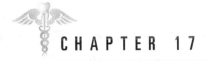

CHAPTER 17

Arthritis

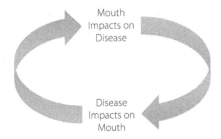

Mouth Impacts on Disease

Disease Impacts on Mouth

What is arthritis? Arthritis is a collection of diseases in which the joints become inflamed. It can be extremely uncomfortable and leads to crippling disability. It is estimated that about 70% of all seventy-year-olds suffer from arthritis, but it can affect children as well as adults. It often starts when we are in our thirties. Quality of life is significantly affected in those with arthritis.

IMPACT OF MOUTH ON ARTHRITIS

There are studies that show a link between oral inflammation and the risk of rheumatoid arthritis. People with gum inflammation are three times more likely to develop arthritis.[67]

---

67 Molitor, J. A. and Majka, D., Unhealthy Gums Linked to Development of Rheumatoid Arthritis. American College of Rheumatology Annual Meeting. Philadelphia, s.n., 2009.

IMPACT OF ARTHRITIS ON THE MOUTH

Those with the condition find it increasingly difficult to carry out effective oral hygiene measures. This is because arthritis affects their manual dexterity.

ROLE OF DENTAL MEDICINE IN ARTHRITIS

Experts in Dental Medicine will help to prevent this condition by eliminating oral inflammation. We also help patients with existing arthritis to maintain healthy mouths by instructing them in techniques and methods that take into account the challenges caused by their manual dexterity.

And once again we can see a vicious circle exists here.

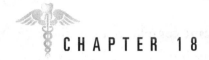

CHAPTER 18

Kidney Disease

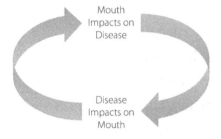

Mouth Impacts on Disease

Disease Impacts on Mouth

What is kidney disease? Approximately one million people in the UK have kidney disease. The role of the kidneys is primarily to remove 'waste' products from our bodies. Without properly functioning kidneys, these toxic substances build up, resulting in death. Kidneys also make red blood cells, which carry oxygen around the body and have a role in maintaining correct blood pressure. Those with kidney failure are often on kidney dialysis. Dialysis is a mechanical system that carries out the removal of the toxic substances.

The kidneys are among the most important organs when it comes to bone metabolism (bone metabolism is the turnover of bone). In the section on osteoporosis, I mentioned that Dental Medicine Experts have knowledge of bone and its metabolism, a natural process which serves to keep the bone alive.

IMPACT OF THE MOUTH ON KIDNEY DISEASE

Kidney failure is one of the significant complications in those who have diabetes, so there is an indirect link between the mouth and kidney disease.

IMPACT OF KIDNEY DISEASE ON THE MOUTH

As teeth are supported by bone, anything that affects bone metabolism can affect the teeth. Kidney disease and the medications used to treat it can cause a number of problems in the mouth including dry mouth, loosening of teeth, and inflammation of the mouth and salivary glands.

If you have kidney disease and are having dental implants to replace missing teeth, it is crucial that your dentist is aware of your medical history. He or she will probably need to consult with your doctor prior to starting treatment.

ROLE OF DENTAL MEDICINE IN KIDNEY DISEASE

We have already seen the role of Dental Medicine in diabetes, and as diabetes is the main cause of kidney failure in the UK, Dental Medicine plays an important role in this disease as well.

We need to take into account the kidney function of those with kidney disease when considering any treatment such as implants. This is another area where Dental Medicine Experts would ideally be involved in the care of the patient.

We therefore recognise a vicious circle exists here.

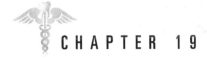

CHAPTER 19

Gastrointestinal Issues

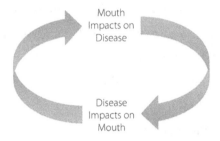

Mouth Impacts on Disease

Disease Impacts on Mouth

What are gastrointestinal issues? This is a collection of conditions that many people have heard of, and even suffered from. It includes indigestion and reflux (sometimes causing pain which is called heartburn; at other times causing no pain at all), but it also includes gastric ulcers which can be fatal if they bleed.

IMPACT OF THE MOUTH ON GASTROINTESTINAL ISSUES

The bacteria that often cause gastric ulcers are called Helicobacter pylori. These bacteria can often be found in the mouth. Someone who has been treated for gastric ulcers may develop them again later due to re-infection by these bacteria.

People who cannot chew properly often swallow food in larger 'lumps', so their stomach and intestines have to work a lot harder to break that food down. This increases risk of indigestion and reflux and is likely to have an effect on the body's ability to take in all the nutrients it needs.

IMPACT OF GASTROINTESTINAL ISSUES ON THE MOUTH

Teeth are 'designed' to undergo normal wear and tear. Excessive wear can occur as a result of acid reflux. Acid from the stomach can soften the surface of the teeth, which will then wear down more rapidly than normal. You may detect this yourself in the later stages as a shortening of the upper front teeth. They may start to chip at the tips (as they get thinner from behind). Sometimes they can appear more translucent/blue in appearance.

Your dentist and doctor will probably need to consult to work out the best way to treat this problem.

A similar process can occur from a regular intake of acidic food or drink such as frequent citrus fruit drinks. However, the parts of the teeth that wear tend to follow a different pattern which a Dental Medicine Expert will be able to identify depending on the source of the acid (e.g. reflux tends to affect the upper molars on the side by the roof of the mouth). It is best to avoid tooth-brushing immediately after an acidic intake. A small piece of cheese can also help neutralise the acids.

ROLE OF DENTAL MEDICINE IN GASTROINTESTINAL ISSUES

As you can see, the mouth plays a role in several gastrointestinal issues. Dental Medicine Experts are always concerned about general heath and are keen to eliminate oral causes. There's a reciprocal impact on the teeth and mouth for some gastrointestinal issues, which means another vicious circle.

IMAGE 1

Dental Medicine Triangle: shows the three cornerstones behind the philosophy of Dental Medicine

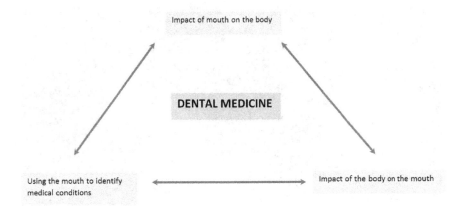

IMAGE 2

The marginal ridge of the tooth, loss of the marginal ridge through decay will significantly affect the ridgity of the tooth

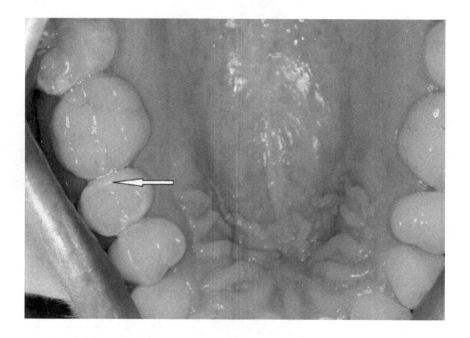

IMAGE 3

An overhanging filling which is impossible to clean effectively

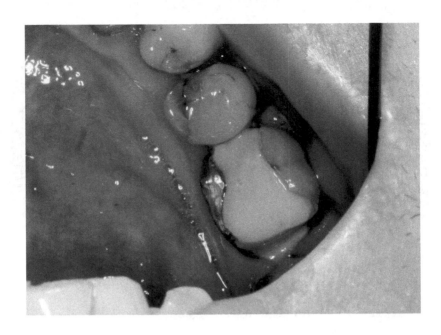

IMAGE 4

An x-ray picture of the tooth in image 3 showing the challenge that such a poorly placed restoration creates for effective cleaning

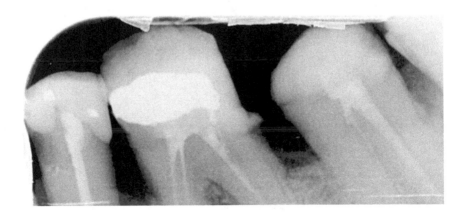

IMAGE 5

A draining infection from a tooth which gave no apparent pain or symptoms

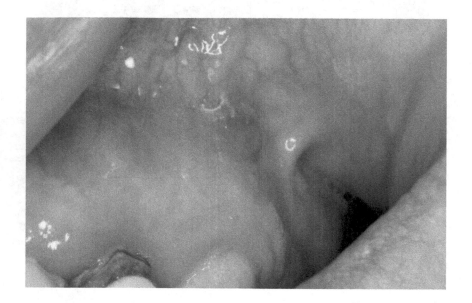

IMAGE 6

An x-ray picture of the tooth from image 5 showing the infection at the top of the root

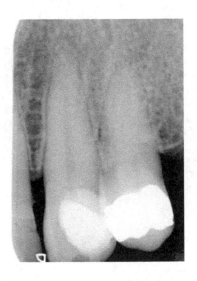

IMAGE 7

An x-ray picture of the tooth from images 5 and 6 showing the root canal filling in the tooth root

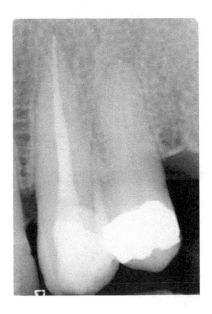

IMAGE 8

A photo of the same tooth from images 5, 6 and 7 showing the draining infection has now resolved following appropriate treatment

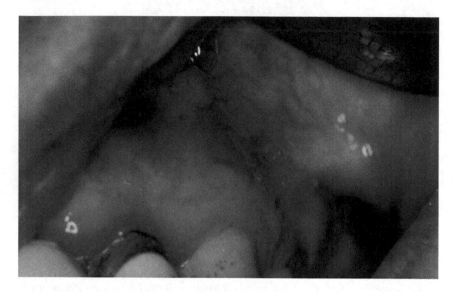

IMAGE 9

An indication of the mechanisms of how inflammation can impact on diabetes and glycaemic control

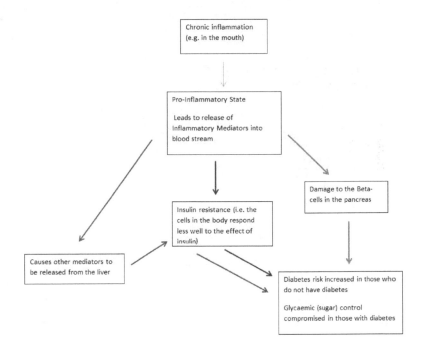

IMAGE 10

A diagram to show atheromatous (arterial) diseases and the conditions it can cause

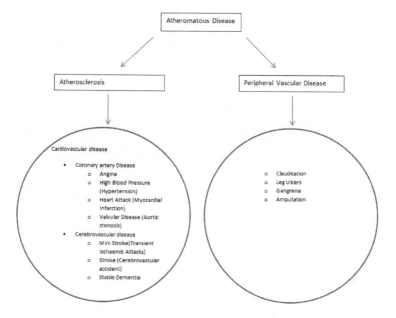

CHAPTER 20

Saliva and Salivary Concerns

Saliva receives its own chapter because its role is often undervalued. I predict that over the next few years saliva will become an essential tool in helping us diagnose dental disease and general health issues. Dentists will have an increasing role to play in this.

Saliva has many roles. It helps start the digestion process when we eat and drink. It lubricates the mouth and protects the soft tissues of the mouth. It also reduces the risk of decay. It carries immune components, so it reduces inflammation in the mouth.

There are two main parts to saliva. The fluid part makes up the majority of saliva, and held within this are proteins and molecules. There is also a mucous part that helps lubricate and protect the mouth.

SALIVA AND DECAY

Decay occurs when bacteria in plaque produce acid which then dissolves the tooth. As this enlarges, a cavity forms. When eating (or even when stimulated by the smell of food), our salivary glands increase the amount of saliva produced. This saliva helps in two ways. It helps clear food from the mouth, therefore reducing the time that bacteria are in contact with the food and reducing the damage they can cause. It also contains bicarbonate (which is produced in increased amounts as the saliva flow increases). Bicarbonate is a buffer. This means it neutralises acid and so helps reduce the damage that the acid will cause to teeth.[68]

We observe that those with reduced salivary flow rates (e.g. after radiotherapy to the salivary glands, or in Sjogren's syndrome, and due to certain drugs) have an increased risk of decay.

SALIVA AND GUM DISEASE

It has been shown that those with gum disease have saliva with a less effective antioxidant effect than the saliva in those who do not have gum disease (antioxidants help reduce the damage caused by sunlight, tobacco, food, etc.) At the moment this situation is a bit 'chicken and egg', as we do not know if the saliva is impacting the gum disease, or if the gum disease is impacting the saliva.[69]

SALIVA AND DIABETES

In the section on diabetes I mentioned that saliva may have a role in reducing the risk of diabetes. Those with diabetes are also more likely to have a dry mouth.

SALIVA AS A DIAGNOSTIC TOOL

There are many benefits to using saliva as a diagnostic tool. It's easily accessible. We've all seen the programmes on TV where they

---

68 Cawson, R. A. and Odell, E. W., *Essentials of Oral Pathology and Oral Medicine*. London: Churchill Livingstone, 1997.

69 Sculley, D. V. and Langley-Evans, S. C., 'Periodontal Disease Is Associated with Lower Antioxidant Capacity in Whole Saliva and Evidence of Increased Protein Oxidation', *Clin. Sci.*, 105/2 (2003), 167–72.

swab someone's saliva for DNA tests. Diagnostic tests can be carried out in much the same way, eliminating the need for taking blood, which can be difficult and unpleasant. Sometimes more saliva is needed and the patient simply drools into a beaker.

I referred earlier to the components of saliva. These come from the 'plasma' part of blood. Therefore saliva contains various proteins at the same level as they are in blood. It is these proteins that can be used as markers. When using saliva as a diagnostic tool, we are looking for the 'markers'. They can be used in both diagnosis and in monitoring the effect of treatment for a range of diseases including cancer, infections, and hereditary conditions. They can also be used to help optimise the amount of medication that is ideal to give someone. The markers measured tend to be specific hormones, specific enzymes, or hereditary material.[70]

SALIVA AND VIRAL INFECTIONS

Saliva can be used to test for HIV (human immunodeficiency virus) with similar accuracy to a blood test.[71]

Saliva can be used to help diagnose viral hepatitis, and can also be used to assess the immunization status of measles, mumps, and rubella.[72]

---

70 Shankar, A. A. and Dandekar, R. C., 'Salivary Biomarkers: An Update', *Dent. Update*, 39/8 (2012), 566–72.

71 Malamud, D., 'Saliva as a Diagnostic Fluid', *Br. Med. J.*, 305 (1992), 207–8.

Gaudette, D. et al., 'Stability of Clinically Significant Antibodies in Saliva and Oral Fluid', *J. Clin. Immunoassay*, 17 (1994), 171–5.

72 Parry, J. V. et al., 'Diagnosis of Hepatitis A and B by Testing Saliva', *J. Med. Virol.*, 28/4 (1989), 255–60.

Thieme, T. et al., 'Determination of Measles, Mumps, and Rubella Immunisation Status Using Oral Fluid Samples', *J. Am. Med. Assoc.*, 272/3 (1994), 219–21.

SALIVA AND MALIGNANCY

Saliva has a broad scope of use in cancer screening. It can be used to detect breast cancer, ovarian cancer, and oral cancer.[73]

SALIVA AND DRUGS

Saliva can be used to measure drug concentrations in the body.[74] It can be used to monitor patient compliance with psychiatric medication[75] and to detect use of illicit drugs including amphetamines, barbiturates, cocaine, benzodiazepines, and opioids.[76]

SALIVA AND SYSTEMIC CONDITIONS

Following a myocardial infarct (heart attack), saliva can be used to help with the diagnosis.[77]

---

73 Streckfus, C. et al., 'A Preliminary Study of CA15-3, c-erbB-2, Epidermal Growth Factor Receptor, Cathepsin-D, and p53 in Saliva among Women with Breast Carcinoma', *Cancer Invest.*, 18/2 (2000), 101–9.

Chien, D. X. and Schwartz, P. E., 'Saliva and Serum CA 125 Assays for Detecting Malignant Ovarian Tumors', *Obstet. Gynecol.*, 75/4 (1990), 701–4.

Tavassoli, M. et al., 'p53 Antibodies in the Saliva of Patients with Squamous Cell Carcinoma of the Oral Cavity', *Int. J. Cancer.*, 78/3 (1998), 390–1.

Mizukawa, N. et al., 'Defensin-1, a Peptide Detected in the Saliva of Oral Squamous Cell Carcinoma Patients', *Anticancer Res.*, 18/6B (1998), 4645–9.

74 Drobitch, R. K. and Svensson, C. K., 'Therapeutic Drug Monitoring in Saliva: An Update', *Clin. Pharmacokinet.*, 23/5 (1992), 365–79.

75 Kaufman, E. and Lamster, A. B., 'The Diagnostic Applications of Saliva: A Review', *Crit. Rev. Oral Biol. Med.*, 13/2 (2002), 197–212.

76 Kidwell, D. A., Holland, J. C., and Athanaselis, S., 'Testing for Drugs Abuse in Saliva and Sweat', *J. Chromatogr. B: Biomed. Sci. Appl.*, 713/1 (1998), 111–35.

77 Floriano, P. N. et al., 'Use of Saliva-Based Nano Biochip Tests for Acute Myocardial Infarction at the Point of Care: A Feasibility Study', *Clin. Chem.*, 55/8 (2009), 1530–8.

Coeliac disease is a condition in which people are not able to eat food with gluten in it. Saliva can be used to detect coeliac and to help monitor how closely patients are sticking to a gluten-free diet.[78]

SALIVA AND AUTO-IMMUNE DISORDERS

Sjogren's syndrome directly affects the salivary glands. It also leads to a release of markers in the saliva, so there is scope for saliva to be used to test for Sjogren's.[79]

SALIVA AND STRESS

There are various markers in saliva that may be useful in helping to diagnose stress.[80]

SALIVA AND ENDOCRINE STATUS

Insulin can be detected in saliva and so can be used to monitor insulin levels in patients with endocrine disorders, such diabetes, or in patients who are at risk of diabetes.[81]

---

78 al-Bayaty, H. F. et al., 'Salivary and Serum Antibodies to Gliadin in the Diagnosis of Celiac Disease', *J. Oral. Pathol. Med.*, 18/10 (1989), 578–81.

Hakeem, V. et al., 'Salivary IgA Antigliadin Antibody as a Marker for Coeliac Disease', *Arch. Dis. Child.*, 67/6 (1992), 724–7.

79 Hu, S. et al., 'Salivary Proteomic and Genomic Biomarkers for Primary Sjogren's Syndrome', *Arthritis Rheum.*, 56/11 (2007), 3588–600.

80 Rohleder, N. et al., 'Psychosocial Stress-Induced Activation of Salivary Alpha-Amylase: An Indicator of Sympathetic Activity?', *Ann. NY Acad. Sci.*, 1032 (2004), 258–63.

Malamud, D., 'Saliva as a Diagnostic Fluid', *Dent. Clin. N. Am.*, 55/1 (2011), 159–78.

81 Marhetti, P. et al., 'Salivary Insulin Concentrations in Type-2 (Non-Insulin-Dependent) Diabetic Patients and Obese Non-diabetic Subjects: Relationship to Changes in Plasma Insulin Levels after an Oral Glucose Load', *Diabetologia.*, 29/10 (1986), 695–8.

So saliva plays an important role on a number of levels and its benefits are often undervalued. Due to the ease of saliva collection, it is likely that its role in medicine will increase significantly in the near future.

CHAPTER 21

Halitosis (Bad Breath)

Halitosis, or bad breath, is a condition that makes people very self-conscious and embarrassed. It is believed about 30–50% of the adult population suffer from it. In many cases it is easy to treat.

There are many potential causes (see list below), but most of the time (in about 85% of cases) the mouth is the cause.[82] Our role as experts in Dental Medicine is to eliminate causes related to the mouth first, and then consult with general medical practitioners/specialists if this does not solve the problem.

CAUSES OF BAD BREATH

There are a number of causes of bad breath:[83]

- oral infection

---

82 Bollen, C.M. L. and Beikler, T., 'Halitosis: The Multidisciplinary Approach', *Int. Jour. Oral Science.,* 4/2 (2012), 55–63.

83 Bollen, C.M. L. and Beikler, T., 'Halitosis: The Multidisciplinary Approach', *Int. Jour. Oral Science.,* 4/2 (2012), 55–63.

Scully, C. and Felix, D. H., 'Oral Medicine—Update for the Dental Practitioner: Oral malodour', *BDJ,* 199/8 (2005), 498–500.

Fedorowicz, Z. et al., 'Mouthrinses for the Treatment of Halitosis', the Cochrane Collaboration, *Cochrane Database of Systematic Reviews,* 4 (Oct. 2008).

Suzuki, N. et al., 'The Relationship between Alcohol Consumption and Oral Malodour', *Int. Dent. Jour.,* 59/1 (2009), 31–4.

- decay
- gum disease
- tongue
- dry mouth
- starvation
- certain foods
- smoking
- alcohol
- some drugs
- disease
- diabetes
- gastrointestinal disease
- liver failure
- kidney failure
- respiratory disease (e.g. nasal sepsis, sinusitis, tonsillitis)
- other

What can you do about it? Clearly with so many causes, the way to help will vary depending on the cause. There are some causes you can manage yourself while others may need professional intervention.

MORNING BREATH

This is probably the most common type of bad breath. During sleep saliva flow is reduced; in addition, many people breathe through their mouths during sleep, which causes dryness. Normally a rinse with fresh water or brushing with a toothbrush and toothpaste will solve the problem.

DRY MOUTH (XEROSTOMIA)

Those who suffer from a reduced salivary flow benefit from regular sips of water and chewing sugar-free gum, or sucking sugar-free sweets, to moisten their mouths and reduce the risk of bad breath.

FOOD

There are a number of foods that cause halitosis, including onions, brussel sprouts, garlic, cabbage, spices, and radish. Also, alcohol and cigarettes are known to affect breath. Simply avoiding these will help. Halitosis caused by food is obviously a temporary problem which stops when the offending items are avoided.

GUM DISEASE

This is one of the main causes. If someone has gum disease that has not been diagnosed, either because they have not been to the dentist for a while, or because their dentist has failed to assess their gum health accurately (remember gum disease almost never causes any problems such as pain), there will be a collection of bacteria which will cause odours to be released. The best way to address this is to have the gum disease treated (and as we see in this book, the results of treatment will benefit much more than your gums and breath).

As a temporary measure, there are ways to help cover up the odour which will be discussed later. To combat gum disease you will need to dedicate time and effort to a daily cleaning regime. While you are waiting for a dental opinion, it's worth starting to clean your teeth, gums, and tongue as well as possible, including the areas between teeth. Daily cleaning has been shown to reduce the risk of halitosis.[84]

DECAY

Cavities in teeth hold a collection of bacteria, feasting off the food and drink that you consume! These bacteria also cause odours to be released and so can cause bad breath. As with gum disease, the best course of action is to have the decay treated.

TONGUE

It is thought that this is one of the major causes of bad breath.[85] The top surface of the tongue is rough and there are lots of hiding places for bacteria. Using a tongue scraper, or simply using a toothbrush to brush the tongue a couple of times a day can help. Some find this makes them gag when they do it, but over time it becomes easier. The aim is to reach as far back as possible, so it is often easier to hold and pull the tongue forward with your free hand whilst cleaning it. A gentle brushing is all that is needed.

OTHER ORAL INFECTIONS

Infections around teeth (particularly wisdom teeth) that are not fully erupted in the mouth, infections following tooth extraction, and infections in areas of oral cancer can all cause bad breath. If you suspect any of these, you should book an appointment immediately.

---

84 Eldarrat, A. H., 'Influence of Oral Health and Lifestyle on Oral Malodour', *Int. Dent. J.*, 61/1 (2011), 47–51.

85 Bollen, C.M. L. and Beikler, T., 'Halitosis: The Multidisciplinary Approach', *Int. Jour. Oral Science.*, 4/2 (2012), 55–63.

In children, the loss of baby teeth and the subsequent emergence of adult teeth often lead to a bout of bad breath. Intervention is rarely needed, unless it is a prolonged problem.

MOUTHWASHES

Mouth washes can help with bad breath. Some just camouflage the odour, while others aim to neutralise it.

A mouthwash containing 0.05% chlorhexedine and 0.05% cetylpyridium chloride and 0.14% zinc lactate significantly reduced halitosis in one study.[86] However, chlorhexedine can cause staining and tongue discolouration.

TOOTHPASTE

Toothpastes containing stannous fluoride, zinc, or triclosan have been shown to have some effect in reducing bad breath.[87]

GASTROINTESTINAL DISEASE

There are studies that show links with halitosis and gastrointestinal disease. They have also shown that by treating the gastric problems, the halitosis improves in a number of patients.[88] However,

---

86 Fedorowicz, Z. et al., 'Mouthrinses for the Treatment of Halitosis', the Cochrane Collaboration, *Cochrane Database of Systematic Reviews,* 4 (Oct. 2008).

87 Bollen, C.M. L. and Beikler, T., 'Halitosis: The Multidisciplinary Approach', *Int. Jour. Oral Science.,* 4/2 (2012), 55–63.

88 Kinberg, S. et al., "The Gastrointestinal Aspects of Halitosis', *Can. J. Gastroenterol.,* 24/9 (2010), 552–6.

there are other studies that question the role of the gastrointestinal tract on halitosis.[89] This is an area of on-going research.

ROLE OF DENTAL MEDICINE IN HALITOSIS

As you can see, the mouth plays a significant role in managing the cause of bad breath in the majority of cases. As Dental Medicine Experts, we are always concerned about general heath, so we are keen to eliminate oral causes. This means that patients can have increased confidence and be less self-conscious, but it also means that potentially life-threatening conditions can be treated.

QUICK TIPS: STEPS TO CONTROLLING BAD BREATH

1. Treat any identifiable causes such as gum disease and decay.
2. Avoid foods that cause bad breath.
3. Avoid habits such as alcohol intake and tobacco use.
4. Brush teeth after meals.
5. Ensure a good oral hygiene regime is carried out regularly.
6. Eat a good breakfast, and eat regular meals including fresh fruit.
7. Use mouthwash twice daily.
8. Clean your tongue (the top surface).
9. Keep your mouth as moist as possible (sugar-free chewing gum or sugar-free sweets, and regular drinks of water can help).
10. Use breath fresheners.

---

89 Bollen, C.M. L. and Beikler, T., 'Halitosis: The Multidisciplinary Approach', *Int. Jour. Oral Science.*, 4/2 (2012), 55–63.

11. If you have dentures, leave them out at night, ideally soaking in an appropriate cleaner.

CHAPTER 22

Snoring and Sleep Apnoea

Snoring is often the butt of jokes and jibes, but it can be an indicator of a serious condition with significant consequences. Did you know 75% of couples regularly sleep in separate rooms? To make matters worse, the vast majority of these couples think their sleeping arrangements are socially unacceptable, so they avoid talking about them openly. Many of them are embarrassed that one, or both, of them snores. As more than 40% of the UK population snore, it's nothing to be embarrassed about, especially since there are things that can be done to help.

A disturbed sleep inevitably impacts on sufferers and their partners' lifestyle. (I will leave it up to you to decide whether it is the snorer or the partner who is the 'sufferer'!)

They often notice that they are less effective at work, have higher stress levels, poorer sex life, and constant daytime sleepiness. Did you know about the danger of accidents at work or the potential to fall asleep at the wheel caused by lack of sleep due to snoring? Worse still, serious health risks are associated with snoring (see below). Snoring is not 'just a noise!'

Snoring is caused by a partial closure of the airway during sleep, due to a relaxation of the muscles in the neck. The vibration of these muscles causes that characteristic sound.

SELF-HELP FOR SNORERS

1. Sew a tennis ball into the back of your pyjamas. This forces you to roll onto your front when you sleep, causing the lower jaw to drop forward, clearing your airway. This technique is a primitive and indirect version of a mandibular advancement device but doesn't work that well.
2. Lose weight. Snoring is more likely if someone is overweight, especially if any of that extra weight is around the neck area. Regular exercise and a healthy diet will help.
3. Lay off the alcohol. Alcohol causes muscles to relax and increases airway obstruction during sleep.

MANDIBULAR ADVANCEMENT DEVICES

Many have tried (or been forced to try) nasal strips, throat sprays, and a whole host of self-help measures. Sadly, the fact is that for most snorers unless the space behind our tongues is opened to allow more air through, these measures offer little relief. A mandibular advancement device works like the tennis ball but in a much more controlled way! It gently positions the lower jaw (i.e. the mandible) forward and opens the airway up. This device needs to be made by someone with a special interest in snoring and sleep apnoea. It takes about two to three months to get used to, but it can help you return to sharing your marital bed. It is the most non-invasive, comfortable, and inexpensive solution available.

If you do snore, a screening process to rule out obstructive sleep apnoea is recommended.

OBSTRUCTIVE SLEEP APNOEA

Some people not only have a partial closure but also stop breathing repeatedly throughout the night. This is obstructive sleep apnoea (OSA), and in severe cases, sufferers spend more than half an hour of their average sleep depriving their bodies of oxygen. They are at higher risk of high blood pressure, stroke, heart failure, heart attacks, diabetes, and depression. It will also affect their daily activity and ability to concentrate, be effective, and be safe.

THE ROLE OF DENTAL MEDICINE IN SLEEP APNOEA AND SNORING

In those who snore and who do not show the signs of sleep apnoea, a simple mandibular advancement system can help.

In those with sleep apnoea or at risk of sleep apnoea, we consult with the sleep clinics to help ensure the best solution is provided. This solution can sometimes be as simple as a mandibular advancement device, but often a combination of lifestyle and intervention solutions are needed.

Dental Medicine Experts are well positioned to be able to discuss these problems with patients and suggest the best course of action.

CHAPTER 23

Oral Lesions: Blisters, Ulcers, Lumps, and Patches

T he list of conditions that can cause blisters, ulcers, lumps, and white and red patches in the mouth is extremely long. It includes recurrent aphthous stomatitis, Behcet's disease, erythema multiforme, ulcerative colitis, Crohn's disease, coeliac disease, lupus, lichen planus, pemphigus vulgaris, pemphigoid, viruses, drug-related reactions, and cancer, to name a few. It is beyond the scope of this book to explain each of them. A large part of the dental undergraduate curriculum is dedicated to enabling dentists to identify the cause, often in liaison with appropriate hospital consultants.

ROLE OF DENTAL MEDICINE IN BLISTERS, ULCERS, LUMPS, AND PATCHES

Our main role is to identify the cause, then to aid in elimination of the cause if possible. If eliminating the cause is not possible we aim to help reduce the impact of the symptoms.

CHAPTER 24

Psoriasis

What is psoriasis? Psoriasis is a condition that affects the skin. It happens when the cells that form the skin are produced too rapidly, leading to overgrowth of the skin, which creates the lesions. The condition is not contagious, and occurs due to faulty signals in the immune system which cause new skin cells to be made too rapidly.

When it flares, it can cause severe itching and pain. Sometimes the skin cracks and bleeds. Psoriasis tends to be a lifelong condition and can cause embarrassment and low self-esteem.

IMPACT OF MOUTH ON PSORIASIS

A study of almost a quarter of a million people has shown that those with gum disease are 54% more likely to get psoriasis.[90]

ROLE OF DENTAL MEDICINE IN PSORIASIS

This research is relatively new. However, if there is a link between gum inflammation and psoriasis, this further reinforces the philosophy behind Dental Medicine and reinforces the benefit of the work that Dental Medicine Experts do.

---

90 Keller, J. J. and Lin, H.-C., 'The Effects of Chronic Periodontitis and its Treatment on the Subsequent Risk of Psoriasis', *Br. J. Dermatol.*, 167/6 (2012), 1338–44.

CHAPTER 25

Drugs and Their Oral Side Effects

T he list of medications which can impact the mouth is extensive and their effects can vary. As you may expect, not all people are affected in the same way. Some may experience major side effects, while others experience none.

DRUGS AND DRY MOUTH

Drugs are the main cause of dry mouth (xerostomia). There are more than 400 medications that are known to cause dry mouth. There are other causes of dry mouth such as diabetes and Sjogren's syndrome. Dry mouth will increase the risk of tooth decay and will decrease the protective role of saliva. We saw earlier that saliva has a cleansing effect, but it also has an anti-inflammatory role. Dryness will increase the chance of developing inflammation in the mouth, and as we know, inflammation which continues long-term is not good. Custom-designed oral hygiene programmes are beneficial to those with dry mouth to help prevent decay and other general health problems.

Although dry mouth from drugs can be a nuisance, normally the benefit of the medication outweighs the discomfort and risks.

Dental Medicine Experts will aim to minimise the impact of dryness on the mouth.

QUICK FACTS: SOME MEDICINES THAT CAUSE DRY MOUTH

- anti-anxiety medication
- Alzheimer's disease medication
- antidepressants
- antihistamines
- anti-nausea medication
- blood pressure medications
- 'cold' cures containing ephedrine
- decongestants
- diuretics
- heart rhythm medication
- inhalers
- Parkinson's disease medication
- seizure medication

DRUGS AND GINGIVAL (GUM) OVERGROWTH

There is a specific form of gingival overgrowth that is caused by particular medications. This is called gingival hypertrophy. It results in the gums enlarging, thus making effective cleaning impossible. Sometimes this overgrowth can completely cover the teeth. In extreme cases surgery is often needed. Patients with this condition will not be able to maintain their mouth easily, so they rely heavily on us to help them. The main causes of drug-related gingival overgrowth are cyclosporine (an immune suppression drug used after organ transplant), phenytoin (an anti-convulsant drug used often in epilepsy) and nifedipine (used to treat high blood pressure).

DRUGS AND DECAY

Many drugs contain sugars. If they are used for long periods of time, they can obviously increase the risk of decay directly. It is worth asking your doctor or pharmacist if sugar-free versions are available.

DRUGS AND FUNGAL INFECTIONS

Certain inhalers used to treat asthma and COPD contain steroids. These steroids are used to suppress your immune system so the effects of the asthma or COPD are lessened. These steroids also affect the oral flora (these are the bugs that normally live in the mouth, predominately bacteria and fungal bugs), and allow some of them to take over. This will lead to oral thrush. If you use inhalers, it is worth rinsing your mouth with water afterwards to reduce the risk of thrush.

DRUGS AND ORAL INFECTIONS

The bugs, or oral flora, that live in the mouth generally live in harmony and keep each other in check. Antibiotics can affect this balance. They kill some of the bacteria and allow the fungi to take over, which can lead to thrush.

DRUGS AND MOUTH ULCERS

Many drugs can cause ulcers and soreness in the mouth. This can often make it more difficult to eat properly and harder to clean effectively. Sometimes we need to work with doctors to find a drug that treats the condition effectively without causing problems in the mouth.

QUICK FACTS: COMMON MEDICATIONS THAT CAUSE MOUTH ULCERS

- nicorandil (used to treat angina)
- beta blockers (used to treat high blood pressure, angina, and abnormal heart rhythms)
- non-steroidal anti-inflammatories such as aspirin and ibuprofen
- oral nicotine replacement therapy
- methotrexate
- penicillin

DRUGS AND MUCOSITIS

Mucositis is inflammation of the lining of the mouth. It is an effect that is normally seen with chemotherapy treatment. It causes pain which can significantly affect eating and drinking as well as effective cleaning.

DRUGS AND TOOTH DISCOLOURATION

Tetracyline antibiotics were used commonly in the 1950s. If used when teeth are developing (including in pregnant mothers), they will affect the child's teeth, leading to bands of discolouration which are very hard to treat. Normally tetracylines are avoided in pregnancy and in those under eight years old.

Other medication (including chlorhexidine mouthwash) can lead to an increase in staining on the teeth. This can usually be polished off by a hygienist.

DRUGS AND LICHENOID REACTIONS

Lichenoid reactions are a type of allergic reaction to drugs which leads to patches appearing on the skin and sometimes in the mouth. The common causes are drugs such as gold (for arthritis), metformin (for diabetes), beta blockers (for high blood pressure and heart conditions) and antimalarials.

DRUGS AND TASTE CHANGES

Many drugs can affect your sense of taste, often leading to a metallic, salty, or bitter taste. The change is usually temporary and returns to normal when the medication is stopped.

QUICK FACTS: COMMON MEDICATIONS THAT CAUSE TASTE CHANGES

- ampicillin, metronidazole, and tetracycline (antibiotics)
- amphoterecin (antifungal)
- chlorpheniramine (antihistamine)
- lithium (antipsychotic)
- bisphosphonates
- diltiazam and enalapril (blood pressure medications)
- gliclazide (diabetes medication)

- nitroglycerin patches (angina medication)
- levodopa (anti-Parkinson's disease)
- carbimazole (thyroid medication)
- nicotine skin patches

ROLE OF DENTAL MEDICINE IN DRUGS AND THEIR SIDE EFFECTS

You have seen that drugs have many effects on the mouth, so there is a significant role that Dental Medicine plays in both minimising their side effects and working with medical teams to care for the patient in the best way.

CHAPTER 26

What Can Be Done to Add 4006 Days to My Life?

W

e now know that there are many diseases with proven links to oral inflammation, and others that are still at the early stages of research. Looking at the developments over the past few years, I wouldn't be at all surprised if the list of diseases with proven links to the mouth continues to grow. This topic is understandably complex since the complex relationships between various diseases make it challenging for the researchers to establish direct links. Some have already been proven; others are yet to be proven or disproved.

The good news is that the ways we can help are much easier to understand. A dentist who wants to help you ensure that your risk of getting any of the above diseases is minimised will do all he or she can to help eradicate any inflammation in the mouth. At the start of this book I mentioned that diseases are 'multifactorial' and that our aim is to reduce your risk of getting these diseases. Removal of oral inflammation is one of the many things we can do. The other factors which help include healthy living, minimising tobacco and alcohol intake, regular exercise, healthy diet, and so on. An in-depth look at all the other aspects is beyond the scope of this book, but it is worth mentioning that all these factors need to be considered. Addressing the mouth in isolation is only one piece of the jigsaw puzzle. Cooperation between you, a Dental Medicine Expert and your medical team will ensure that you get to complete the jigsaw.

If you can only do one thing right now to reduce your chance of getting these diseases, for example, ensuring that your mouth is not impacting the risk, that's better than doing nothing, since you are removing some of the risk. Remember that disease is multifactorial. So, by reducing or removing any of the risk factors, you have taken a positive step to decrease the risk of getting the disease. If you already have any of the medical conditions in this book (or maybe another medical condition that may have a link which is yet to be found), you can improve your ability to manage and control that condition. So, take control of your health and start to invest in your own future. Perhaps start that daily run/walk, modify your diet so that you are getting a good balance of nutrients, or arrange the visit to the dentist that you have been putting off. Each step will help you on the way to a long and healthy life.

Remember there are additional FREE resources available at www.4006days.com; you will need the following code to access the resources (not case sensitive): hgy4006jujth

About 75% of deaths per year in the UK are due to atheromatous disease, cancer, and respiratory disease, and we have seen that the mouth is linked to all of them. It makes sense to ensure that your mouth is not increasing the risk of any of these conditions.[91]

So, how did I calculate that taking steps to improve the health of your mouth can extend your life by 4006 days? I did some research into the average life expectancies of people with various diseases and compared them to the current average life expectancy which is 85-89

---

91 Office for National Statistics, 'Deaths by Underlying Cause', <http://www.ons.gov.uk/ons/rel/vsob1/mortality-statistics--deaths-registered-in-england-and-wales--series-dr-/2010/stb-deaths-by-cause-2010.html#tab-Deaths-by-underlying-cause>.

years in the UK (2010 statistics). As we have seen, these diseases are influenced by the mouth. By ensuring a healthy mouth, you can reduce the risk of getting those diseases, or reduce the impact of them if you already have them.

I accept that this calculation does not stand up to strict mathematical scrutiny and that statistics are not available for all conditions. Additionally the degree to which a disease is controlled has an extremely significant impact. I had to use a little poetic licence, but the principle is sound:

Disease	Average Reduction in Life Span (years)
Diabetes Type 1	20
Diabetes Type 2	10
Atherosclerotic Disease	6
High Blood Pressure	5
COPD	6
Emphysema	24
Cancer	8
Smoking	10
Average	4006 days

If you wish to see a dentist who has the same philosophy as I do and who views his/her patients' mouths as an integral part of their overall health, you need to look no further than www.dentalmedicine.co.uk and click on the 'Find a Dentist' link.

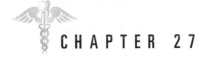

CHAPTER 27

What Can You Do At Home?

You can access the additional resources that are available only to readers of this book. Go to www.4006days.com; you will need the following code to access the resources (not case sensitive): hgy4006jujth

There are a number of other things you can do that will help, but I must introduce a disclaimer here. The only way I can give you advice is to carry out an assessment of your mouth and then offer specific advice based on the findings. I cannot emphasise enough how important it is to have a professional involved in your oral care. With that said, there are some fundamental things that most people should be doing at home.

TOOTHBRUSH

This is top of the list because, for adults, it is the most important thing you can do yourself. The main area where inflammation occurs is around the gums. A toothbrush's main role is to clean the gums where they meet the teeth. You should also brush the teeth. Always spend a good two to three minutes. However, if you have a lot of restorations or have had gum disease in the past, it is likely that you may need to take longer, with a good quality brush. Ensure you get to all areas including the difficult areas! Use of a timer is often helpful. Disclosing tablets or solutions can also help you see areas where your brushing is being effective, and areas where you may need some extra work. These can normally be purchased from dental practices or pharmacies.

A toothbrush typically lasts two months or so. However, those with a heavy hand may find that theirs do not last that long.

Which type of brush—soft versus hard bristles? As we want the bristles to work their way under the gum line to clean there, it is best to use a soft-bristled toothbrush as the soft bristles can do this more easily.

Which type of brush, electric versus manual? It's never a case of one size fits all. If you prefer to use a manual toothbrush and it is effective, there would be little benefit in trying to change it. Electric toothbrushes are definitely easier for many people, and many feel that their teeth are cleaner when compared to using a manual toothbrush. I always advise some caution with electric toothbrushes. They are not quicker; you still need to be meticulous in ensuring the bristles reach all parts of the gums and teeth.

There is evidence that an electric toothbrush with a rotating oscillation action (i.e. the head moves in one direction and then the other) provides better long-term and short-term protection against gum inflammation.[92]

One of the other roles of the toothbrush is to 'transport' toothpaste to the teeth.

Having to brush your teeth may seem like a hassle, particularly when you are rushed or tired, but the desire to eliminate any inflammation from your gums so you can reap the oral and general health benefits will, hopefully, encourage you to keep this good habit. Most people need to brush twice a day; others may need to do it more fre-

---

92   Robinson, P. et al., 'Manual Versus Powered Toothbrushing for Oral Health. Cochrane Database of Systematic Reviews', *Cochrane Database of Systematic Reviews,* issue 2 (2005).

quently depending on other factors such as past disease (both mouth disease and general health status).

TOOTHPASTE

The main benefit of toothpaste is as a fluoride delivery system. I recognise there are differing opinions on fluoride and without wishing to open up the fluoride debate, the benefits of fluoride in reducing the risk of tooth decay has such a wealth of evidence supporting it that the majority of dental professionals accept it as fact. We accept that there are risks with high fluoride doses, but the same is true with high doses of vitamins A, B12, D, K, iron, calcium, and folic acid. The area of debate is whether small doses are harmful. I have looked at the evidence for and against this argument, and my feeling is that the known benefit of fluoride outweighs the possible risks. Putting my money where my mouth is, I use fluoride toothpaste as do my two young sons.

There are other benefits of toothpaste such as removal of staining, freshening of breath, and reduction of tartar build up.

You should use toothpaste every time you brush your teeth.

INTERDENTAL CLEANING

The toothbrush is important in cleaning the gums in particular. However, a toothbrush, no matter how good, and how good your technique, will not clean effectively in between the teeth. This area is called the interdental or interproximal area and accounts for a large portion of the gums (around 35%) where inflammation can occur. Many people find cleaning interdental areas difficult and so often do not bother. However, they are putting themselves at risk of both gum disease and general health issues. It's a bit like doing the washing up after dinner, but only cleaning half the crockery, and putting the rest away dirty!

There are various methods available for cleaning in between teeth including floss, flossettes (i.e. floss held on a plastic holder), and interdental brushes and sticks. Some people need to use a combination of methods depending on their manual dexterity, how easily they can open their mouths, their gag reflex, the restorations they have had previously, any spacing or crowding, and any gum recession. Often over time the techniques used need to evolve as the mouth changes.

If you find interdental cleaning difficult (especially if that means that you do not do it), seek professional help to see if there are alternative techniques suitable for you.

I would recommend that most people carry out interdental cleaning twice a day. Similar to effective tooth brushing, it will take time to do it well, but it's an investment worth making, don't you think?

MOUTHWASH

I often recommend a fluoride mouthwash to those who are susceptible to decay. It is best to use it at a different time than fluoride toothpaste, simply because the benefit will be greater.

There's a lot of advertising on the benefits of antibacterial mouthwashes and their effects on gum disease. I would really like to emphasise that the most important factors in preventing inflamed gums are the tooth brushing technique and the interdental cleaning. Do antibacterial mouthwashes have an effect? Possibly, but if they do, it is a small effect when compared to the daily cleaning regime.

There is certainly no harm in using them; I often recommend them to those who are susceptible to gum disease or have a relevant medical condition. I prefer to adopt a 'belts-and-braces' approach for these people.

SELF-INSPECTION

If you are not seeing a dentist regularly, you should get to know the inside of your mouth. Have a look around at the inside of the cheeks, the roof of the mouth, the tongue (especially underneath and on the sides), and the floor of the mouth. If you notice something that wasn't there before, or there's something on one side that isn't on the other side, get it checked out. Any ulcers or lumps or bumps that do not disappear within two to three weeks should be checked out by a dentist.

If you see a dentist regularly, he or she should be checking these areas for you (and if not, ask why).

The main thing we are looking for is any sign of a lesion that is, or may lead to, oral cancer. Early detection means the survival rate of more than five years is almost three times better than if the cancer is detected late. Some lesions that have the potential to turn into cancer (so called pre-cancerous lesions) can be removed and cancer can be prevented completely.

DIET

There is already a chapter in this book on diet, so here I will just emphasise that diet has an effect on the mouth and general health.

Diet and decay are closely related. Many people think that sugary foods cause decay. I lost count many years ago of the number of times people have said, "I can't understand why I have decay as I don't eat a lot of sweets". I really must emphasise that most food and drink contains sugar. The bacteria which cause decay only need a MINISCULE amount of sugar to feed on. It is this process that causes decay.

As an example and not a recommendation: It is better (for your teeth, not your waistline) to eat a large bar of chocolate in a single sitting than take one small square of chocolate and nibble every fifteen minutes through the day.

The most important fact when considering diet and decay is the FREQUENCY with which sugars come into contact with the mouth, not the AMOUNT of sugar. You can identify sugars in the ingredients as they finish with the letters 'ose', for example, sucrose and glucose. However, take care as sometimes starch turns into sugar when food is processed, and drying foods like fruit releases sugar in the drying process.

DENTURE CARE

If you have dentures, I presume that your dentist gave you instructions on how to care for them. There are different types of dentures and they need different methods of care.

Dentures can cause a number of issues:

1. They can lead to fungal infections. This is more common in older dentures. The bugs that cause the infection sit on the surface of the denture, and because the dentures rest against the gums/soft tissues, they cause the tissues to become inflamed. Dentures can also lead to cracking and soreness at the corners of the mouth. It's worth noting that these fungal infections from dentures are never

painful when just affecting the areas in the mouth. If you develop cracking at the corners of the mouth, that can be uncomfortable. In both situations inflammation occurs. The treatment depends on a number of factors, and so if you notice any redness under your denture, it needs to be looked at. The most common place for the problem to occur is under the fitting surface of a top denture, but this will be a tricky area for you to see yourself.

- Following a good cleaning regime will reduce the risk of fungal infections.

2. Dentures can cause accelerated bone loss. This is worse if your denture moves or rocks about, it will be putting excessive pressure on the bone under the gum, causing it to literally be eaten away.

- If you had a denture that used to fit well and now is loose or moving, it really should be checked out by a dentist.

3. We saw earlier that your chewing ability can influence the risk of dementia.

- If you find that you cannot chew harder foods, perhaps it's time for a dentist to have a look. These changes tend to occur gradually, so you may not notice a difference unless you really think about what you can eat now compared to, say, five years ago.

We know that about 40% of the UK population do not visit a dentist regularly, so if that is you, I hope this section has helped a bit in ensuring that you can do a great deal at home to maintain a healthy mouth. I would like to encourage you to visit a good dentist regularly, as professional intervention will really accelerate the benefits you receive for your general health. I know there are many reasons why people do not go: some are too anxious; for some it's a financial issue; and for others it has more to do with convenience and time. If you are nervous, some dentists are experienced in dealing with dental anxiety and will be empathetic to your needs. If the issue is cost or time, I hope that one of the benefits you get from this book is seeing that regular dental care is an investment in your health rather than a cost.

Some people feel they are 'too old' to get their mouths and teeth fixed. They think they will not live long enough to reap the benefits. Unfortunately, because of the links between oral and general health, this becomes a self-fulfilling prophecy. I often find that those who do live a long life despite poor oral health struggle to adapt to changes in their mouths and regret not taking earlier intervention.

CHAPTER 28

What Can My Dental Team Do?

....

WARNING: This chapter should not be read by dentists who act unethically or who do not want to provide up to date care for their patients.

....

"Well, all dentists receive the same training, so there should be no difference, right?" Unfortunately the dental profession is not exempt from those who are in it for the wrong reasons. Whilst most dentists are ethical and will provide the best care they can, there are some who either choose not to or who simply do not know how.

I feel there are two situations that you need to avoid:

1. A dentist who is not ethical. I discuss in the next section that there are different ways of treating patients' mouths and an unethical dentist who uses the wrong treatment, or poor quality treatment, can negatively impact your mouth and your general health. How do you know if you have an unethical dentist? I admit it can be difficult to tell. I advise you use your own judgment and instincts here.

2. A dentist who is not up to date. To me, this is all about passion. If you are passionate about something, you will put in the effort to do it well and be sure you are up to date. The techniques, materials, and procedures we use are constantly changing. There's a lot of research that goes into improving the quality and success of dental care, and so what was considered appropriate historically is not what is deemed to be 'best practice' now. I'm not referring to fads and fashions (which do occur in dentistry), but solid research that shows a proven benefit of one technique or material over another. Sometimes this can result in a 180° turnaround in working practice.

Here are a couple of examples: Historically it was thought that if a dentist spotted something that could have been decay (i.e. a suspicious area on a tooth, but not definite decay) the recommendation was to drill it out, then drill away a healthy border around it and fill the hole. Our understanding of the decay process has changed significantly, and we now know that it is reversible (within limits). Now we monitor these areas and use a preventative package to try and achieve reversal. This is one of the reasons why many people had lots of fillings in the past, and now many of the younger generations often have mouths with no fillings.

Gum disease used to be called pyorrhoea. It was believed that it was untreatable. Many have had all their teeth removed and dentures made (often in their early twenties, sometimes as a birthday present—Happy Birthday!). Pregnancy was often the trigger for a full mouth extraction procedure. We know that during pregnancy, existing inflammation of the gums often worsens. We also know that gum disease can be treated. The real shame is that most of these people had a problem that was likely to be completely reversible.

How far back in history are we talking about? Certainly within the memory of many of you reading this book.

So how do you know if your dentist lacks the passion to stay up to date? Again I admit it's hard to know. Perhaps show him or her this book. If your dentist is interested, that suggests he or she is passionate about doing his or her best. If your dentist tries to fob you off, perhaps with a 'Well, I'm only here to look after teeth' . . . I'll leave you to reach your own conclusion!

All dentists in the UK have to attend a certain amount of training each year in order to maintain their registration. A dentist who chooses to do a lot more than this 'basic requirement' is demonstrating that they are passionate about delivering better care and better quality dentistry.

I'm passionate that you find out what impact the mouth plays on general health. I'm also passionate that we, in the dental profession, look after patients who place their trust in us. If patients choose to use the dentists who share this philosophy, the others will have to change and stop offering inferior care.

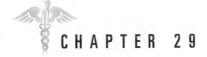
The Way We Look After Patients Will Affect Their Mouths and Their Health

Here I will introduce you to a selection of dental procedures. I'll briefly explain what each is and what each aims to achieve. We can then see why there is a difference in a dentist whose philosophy is about providing great care, such as a Dental Medicine Expert, and a dentist who is unethical or not up to date.

EXAMINATION

"An exam is a check-up is an inspection, right?"

The answer will probably surprise you: No, there is a large difference between what many dentists do and what they can and should be doing.

HISTORY BEHIND A CHECK-UP

A dental exam, or a 'check-up', typically involves the dentist just checking for decay/broken teeth. Remember that there was a time when the profession's understanding of disease processes was very limited, and technology did not allow us to provide the level of care that we now can. Prevention was not really a consideration. If a tooth had a hole, it would either be extracted or repaired with an amalgam filling. Nowadays there could be fifteen to twenty options available for that same tooth.

QUICK FACTS: PREVENTION AND MINIMALLY INVASIVE DENTISTRY

Minimally invasive dentistry is accepted as best practice and this is often made most effective by early intervention when appropriate. We saw in Chapter 6 that the benefits of prevention are significant in terms of cost saving, minimising damage to teeth and so also to general health. Minimally invasive dentistry is not quite as ideal as prevention, but as it preserves more of the natural tooth than 'traditional dentistry' then it's really the next best thing.

The best way to think about prevention and minimal intervention is as a linear scale. With prevention being the preferred option. We always want to choose the most viable option nearest the top of my list below. One major challenge is that in order to do this we need to identify disease in its earliest stages, i.e. when it gives no symptoms at all, or perhaps just very mild symptoms.

THE SCALE OF PREVENTION

Primary prevention: The aim of primary prevention is to prevent the disease occurring in the first place. This is always the best option.

Secondary prevention: The aim of secondary prevention is to identify disease or disease risk very early and then change habits, behaviours or environment to enable the disease to reverse. This means actual intervention is not needed.

Minimal Intervention: Once disease is past the point where secondary prevention will be effective, the aim is to remove the disease whilst preserving as much of the original structure as possible. With teeth, our aim is to preserve enamel and dentine as much as we can.

Traditional Dentistry: This is where the other options are not suitable so traditional dentistry is then needed.

Gum disease was never really diagnosed, particularly in the early stages (which normally give no symptoms). When it was diagnosed by chance, extraction was the only option. If it was not diagnosed at one check-up, it might have been picked up later. The outcome was the same: extraction. There was no understanding that gum disease has an impact on general health. There are many other extremely important aspects of the mouth that are not considered at all with a check-up.

So a 'check-up' worked fine back then, but in recent times the good old check-up just doesn't cut the mustard any more. I would like to be able to say that this is a just a historical thing, but unfortunately it is still the case in a lot of dental practices. I'm not sure why they do not want to provide optimal care, maybe laziness or apathy. Perhaps they are just not up to date on what can be done.

A Dental Medicine Expert, as you would imagine, does not operate like this. I recommend that practices stop offering check-ups. Instead, I recommend a Healthy Mouth Review.

WELCOME TO THE HEALTHY MOUTH REVIEW

What is a Healthy Mouth Review (HMR)? Well, it isn't a check-up by another name.

An HMR is a comprehensive assessment of ALL aspects of the mouth that help us diagnose disease (even in the early stages), identify areas where problems may be about to develop, and look at the impact of the mouth on overall well-being and health. If we want to prevent problems from worsening (e.g. gum disease), we had better pick the problems up at the earliest opportunity.

Let's look at all the parts of the HMR. I use a HMR which is comprised of seventeen parts (when compared to just one or two for a check-up). This is what I am looking for:

- decay/broken teeth
- hidden (symptom free) infections from teeth
- periodontal/gum disease
- soft tissue/cancer screening in the mouth/fungal infection assessment
- face and neck assessment for any signs of melanoma or basal cell carcinomas (rodent ulcers)
- neck assessment for any lymphadenopathy (changes in lymph nodes that may indicate some hidden disease such as cancer)
- pain/sensitivity
- cosmetics
- tooth wear and cracks
- chewing ability
- bite
- jaw joints

- orthodontics
- saliva levels/salivary glands
- general health status
- Dental Medicine (i.e. all of the content in this book)
- specific diabetes screening

I often see new patients who have never had their gums assessed, and we find they have undiagnosed gum disease. Some have been seeing their last dentist for many years. These dentists often fall into the category above of not being up to date. It's embarrassing for us to let these patients know that our profession has failed them, and it is obviously very upsetting for them. So I hope you can see that if we follow the philosophy behind Dental Medicine, we need to offer so much more than a check-up. I would never go for a check-up. Give me a Healthy Mouth Review please.

FILLINGS

I can hear you asking yourself now, is this guy for real? 'A filling is just a filling, right?' You should go and have a look again at Images 3 and 4. The day I do a filling like this is the day I hang up my gloves! When presented with a cavity in a tooth, I would be able to get a filling in that tooth in a few minutes if I chose to do so. The patient is unlikely to know anything as it wouldn't hurt. It would probably look OK in the mirror, and the patient could bite on it. However, this is what I want my filling to achieve:

- I want it to be sealed to prevent bacteria from getting underneath.
- I want it to be long lasting.

- I want it to be aesthetically pleasing.
- I want the tooth to not be sensitive afterwards.
- I want to protect the nerve in the tooth from death.
- I want to increase the strength of the rest of the tooth.
- I want the restoration to be efficient at chewing food.
- I want it to feel like a tooth against the tongue and cheeks.
- I want to eliminate food traps.
- I want it to be smooth, so bugs and plaque can be more easily cleaned off.

In order to achieve these things, I ensure that I am meticulous about many things such as moisture control, having the margin (i.e. where the filling meets the tooth) as flush as possible, and spending time sealing the filling into the tooth. Essentially I am trying to restore the original anatomy (the shape and position) of the tooth. Teeth have evolved over thousands of years to have a particular shape to them as this affects their efficiency. Shouldn't we, as dentists, try to replicate this?

So even though I could place a filling quickly, I choose not to as I would rather provide an excellent restoration that will achieve as many of these ideal qualities as possible. We often use the term 'technique sensitive'. Fillings are highly sensitive to the technique used.

CROWNS/INLAYS/ONLAYS

These are normally used when a filling cannot achieve the ideal qualities listed previously. Most people know what a crown is. It is often called a 'cap'. It sits over the top of the tooth and is cemented on. An inlay is a filling that is made by a technician and fits into a cavity in the tooth. An onlay sits over just the top (i.e. biting) aspect of a tooth. The ideal qualities for a crown/inlay/onlay are the same as for a filling. The other variable in the procedure is that there is a technician (or a machine that makes crowns) involved.

This means that dentists need to somehow get an accurate record of the tooth to the technician (or the machine), and this involves some extra processes. Those processes typically involve taking an impression. The technician makes a model of your tooth from this which he or she uses to create a custom-made restoration for the tooth. There are good technicians and bad technicians. Some have the same philosophy that I do and want to provide excellent restorations that allow us to achieve as many of the ideal qualities as possible. I could send my impressions to China and get the restoration made for minimal cost, but have they used tried and tested materials? Have they been meticulous about creating a restoration that seals well? If I were to use a technician I do not know, it's likely that a different technician would do the work each time, so there would be no relationship between the technician and me, and so no accountability. Does this make a difference to the quality of work? I strongly believe it does. I choose to use the services of technicians I can speak to and who I know will be providing the quality of work that I demand.

There is significant variation in the materials and techniques used for taking impressions, so again we can choose to use the best, or we can choose to use something that is just OK. You wouldn't know, as you would still get a restoration of the tooth, but if we have failed to get an accurate impression, your risk of decay, gum inflammation, and general health problems is increased. How would you know? Well, the scary thing is that you often wouldn't.

On a side note, when making fixed bridges (i.e. ones that are not taken out of the mouth), we need to follow the same principles as outlined above.

IMPLANTS

Implants are typically small titanium rods which replace the root of the tooth, and a restoration (crown/bridge/denture) is placed on top.

The benefits of implants to replace missing teeth are huge. They are independent of the other teeth and so do not risk damaging them (a bridge could damage them, and a denture could as well). Patients often feel that implants are like their normal teeth.

I referred earlier to a filling and crown as aiming to restore the anatomy of the tooth, but the filling, or crown, needs something to stick to and when the tooth is missing, there is nothing there. Enter the 'implant'. Implants also aim to restore the anatomy and are very good at doing this. This is one of the reasons why they have such a good success rate. They also help with chewing ability (see references earlier to dementia risk), reducing the wear and tear on other teeth (so reducing the risk of breakages, etc.), and holding the teeth around them in their correct position, thereby reducing the risk of decay, gum disease, and overloading. Unlike any other replacements for missing teeth, implants also preserve the bone.

When placing implants, consideration of your general health is paramount. My implant training was very much centred on the philosophy of ensuring that general health was optimised before going ahead and placing implants. My understanding of these principles has meant that I can often avoid running into complications that would otherwise be a major headache for both the patient and the dentist.

Implants are a reliable and predictable way to replace missing teeth. They have an excellent success record. However, there are risks; if not handled correctly, they can fail or create problems. So if you are thinking about having implants, read on. As a dentist who has had to fix problems created by others who have placed implants, I would like to share the benefit of my experience with you. There are many excellent dentists out there, and they provide excellent quality dentistry treatment I would be more than happy to have in my mouth. They want to provide dentistry that will be functioning perfectly many years down the line. Unfortunately there are some who do not operate in this way, and they provide poor quality dentistry, be it through poor planning, lack of experience, or just cutting corners. I hope by reading this, you will be in the position to ask the right questions so you can be sure you end up being treated by one of the great dentists.

IS IT BETTER TO LEAVE THE GAP?

I do not want to scare you away from having implants. If done correctly, they are absolutely brilliant at filling gaps. Often patients feel they are better than their natural teeth. They are far superior to dentures, bridges supported by natural teeth, and better than the gap. The ideal time to have an implant is normally within a few months after the tooth has been removed. After this time, the bone in the area where the gap is will gradually disappear, making it harder to restore the space satisfactorily.

A gap which is not filled will lead to increased wear and tear on the remaining teeth. Remember the section, "What role can oral health play"? We looked at just how hard our teeth are made to work. Missing teeth simply increase this workload, which can trigger a succession of other teeth problems leading to further treatment or more extractions.

Gaps also mean the neighbouring teeth and the opposing teeth gradually move out of their correct position and are subject to increased wear and tear since teeth that are not in their correct position can become overloaded more easily, as well as increase the risk of decay and gum disease.

These are the things I think all patients should be aware of when considering implants:

1. Who has made the implant?

There used to be just a handful of implant manufacturers; now there are hundreds. Much of the research into what makes an implant successful in the long term has been carried out by these earlier man-ufacturers. Many of the new systems have not stood the test of time. It will be of little surprise that the newer systems are often cheaper. So is there a risk in using implants that do not have a track record? My feeling is that it's impossible to know. They may even be better than the older systems over a long period of time. However, I personally would only accept a system that has a good track record. I would not want to be a guinea pig. So be sure to ask any dentist thinking of putting an implant in your mouth how long the system he uses has been around. If it's been around for a number of years, it stands to reason that it is OK (otherwise dentists would not use it and the company would cease to exist). My advice is to not let your dentist use your mouth as a testing ground for implants, even if it does save a few hundred pounds per implant. This is a false economy.

2. Surgeon's experience and training

You probably will be surprised to know that a dentist can buy the kit and place an implant in your mouth with no actual training. If something were to go wrong he or she would be in a lot of trouble. However, this would all be after the event. Fortunately this situation is now changing. Many dentists who place implants have chosen to put themselves through rigorous and costly training in order to be able to deliver implant care of high quality. Soon we will reach a time when dentists have to have formal training and then work with a mentor until they have the knowledge and experience to be able to deliver implant care independently. We are not there yet. So ask your dentist what courses he or she has been on. Beware, though. Some courses are 'weekend crash courses' that require no examination at the end. Often the 'experience' is watching someone else do the treatment or placing an implant in a 'plastic jaw'. This is nothing like real life. So I would want to know how long their course ran for, whether they had an examination (otherwise, everyone would 'pass'), and what experience they have had since their training.

The success rate of implants is very high, particularly in the shorter term. This does mean that relatively inexperienced practitioners can often 'get away with it', but their chance of success is more a reflection of the compatibility of implants with the patient than the expertise of the practitioner.

If you do not feel a dentist is competent enough to provide the care you deserve, walk away; it's just not worth the risk.

I would be happy being treated by a 'trainee' who is supervised/assisted by a mentor, as that means I would be receiving care from two professionals who are enthusiastic about providing me with good implants.

3. Restorative dentist: experience + training

There are two parts to an implant: the implant itself, which sits in the bone, and the restoration on top, typically a crown, bridge, or denture. In the same way that I would want someone with suitable experience placing an implant in my mouth, I would also want the person placing the restoration to have training and experience SPE-CIFICALLY IN RESTORING IMPLANTS. All dentists, in theory, can do this, but if the restoration is not correct, it will either fail, or worse still, cause the implant to fail, often leading to a very difficult situation to rectify. Again, I would urge you to ask what training your dentist has had in restoring implants. The 'crash courses' I referred to earlier often do not give any training on the restorative aspect, just a quick reference to it at some point. As I said, the RESTORATION CAN CAUSE THE IMPLANT TO FAIL, so exercise caution.

Would you expect to pay more for an implant from someone who has spent tens of thousands of pounds on training himself or herself to a high level to ensure the treatment you receive is excellent? I would, and again, I think a saving of a few hundred pounds is a false economy.

4. Sterilisation

I have spent a long time researching this, and I can find no reliable evidence that placing implants under a 'sterile' environment affects the success rate. This is most likely because no dentist who is following best practice guidelines would be able to carry out a study. Can you imagine a study in which, in half of our cases, we used optimal sterile practice, in the other half we did not? The study would not (and quite rightly) pass an ethics committee's approval. So does it make a difference? We know that an infection is bad news for an implant. Most that are infected in the early stages will fail. If we operate in a sterile set-up and the risk of infection is reduced, it stands to reason that it is beneficial. So again, I would advise that you check to see if your dentist turns his surgery into a 'mini operating theatre' to carry out implant placement. Walk away if he or she does not. (I can guarantee that dentists having an implant themselves would insist on these measures). How much does it cost to set up like this? Well, to do it properly, it costs from £100 to £200 per case (depending on a few factors). Obviously there is scope for a bit of money saving if these best practice protocols are not followed. But is it worth it?

5. Complications: Does your dentist have any experience in managing them?

Implants are great as they have a very high success rate. The problem is if yours is one of the few that does develop a problem, who is going to sort it out? If your dentist does not have experience in dealing with complications, how is he or she going to deal with your implant complications if you should have them? I feel there are two answers that are acceptable. The first is that your dentist does have experience, often because your dentist deals with other dentists' complications. A failing implant is often difficult to manage. Many times we can salvage it and turn it into a success, but it's not easy, and it's not quick. The other answer I would accept is that your dentist works closely with a colleague who does have experience at handling complications. It would be worth finding out how close that colleague is geographically!

6. Specialist

I sometimes see dentists advertise themselves as specialists in implants/implantology. In the UK there is no such thing. To use the term 'specialist' you need to be on the General Dental Council's specialist register FOR THAT SPECIFIC SPECIALITY. At present there is no implant specialty, so it's impossible to be on a list that does not exist. This is a marketing scam and dentists who claim such a speciality are in breach of regulations that they should be following. If they are prepared to lie about this, what else are they prepared to lie about? Walk away now!!!!

7. Bone grafting: Does your dentist have enough experience?

Even with the best planning in the world, sometimes Mother Nature throws us a curve ball, and what we find at the time of surgery is not what we expected. Inadequate amount of bone is the main problem that could occur. At this stage there are three options:

- Try placing an implant to 'see if it works'. This is not ideal.
- Abandon the treatment. This does you no favours.
- Do something that allows us to place an implant at a later date. By this I mean a bone manipulation process such as bone augmentation.

The ability to do the latter really comes back to experience. So, you really want to know if the surgeon will leave you in the same situation should this problem be discovered (not ideal), or if the surgeon will do something to enable you to have implants later on. My philosophy is that each time I carry out surgery on a patient, I should improve the situation, not to leave the patient in the same situation or worse.

8. Technician

Earlier I advised you that a dentist who does not place the crown on top of the implant correctly can cause failure of the crown or the implant (or both!) The crown (or bridge or denture) is made by a technician, so again, the technician needs to have knowledge and experience of providing restorations for implants. This is why it is worth asking your dentist about the technician's experience.

9. Medical considerations

When placing implants, we are manipulating the natural bony healing processes to our advantage. Many medical conditions will influence this healing process, so, in order to manipulate it, we need to have knowledge of the process and of how medical conditions can influence it. This will come down to the dentist's training. I sometimes make requests for medical investigations and work with general medical practitioners/consultants prior to placing implants. This allows us to ensure the bone healing process is happening normally before we try to manipulate it to our advantage.

10. Overseas: 'dental tourism'

There are many overseas options for having implants. My advice: DON'T DO IT. I really cannot emphasise enough that the potential cost savings are far outweighed by the higher complication rate. Some of the worst cases that I have been involved in 'repairing' come from dental tourism. There's a reason why it's cheap: it's not regulated and involves cheap materials, cheap laboratories, lack of attention to detail, poor planning, and no follow-up.

11. Guarantee

Ask what guarantee your implants have. Consider taking out an insurance policy to help cover any costs incurred should your implant develop a problem. Most dentists with lots of experience will have a policy that allows you to get such coverage.

12. Can it be done on the 'cheap'?

Yes. Can it be done well on the cheap, and take into account all the above factors? No. The investment required for training and using a good quality technician, proper sterilisation processes, and an implant from a manufacturer with a track record have to be incorporated into the fee you pay. If it's done on the cheap, a corner has to be cut somewhere. I think you will agree the savings are not worth the risks?

Once again, implants have the potential to be a long-lasting and superior solution to missing teeth. They can improve your oral health, reduce the amount of dental treatment you need in the future, and benefit your general health. The treatment needs to be carried out by someone who has the necessary experience and ability to pay attention to detail.

ROOT CANAL TREATMENT

Ah, the dreaded root canal treatment! A favourite of dental jokes and films! Just to set the record straight: Root canal treatment should not hurt. If it does, the dentist needs to stop and either give more anaesthetic or dress the tooth with a sedative dressing to reduce the inflammation and then try again another time.

The root canal is a tunnel (or tunnels) in the tooth where the nerve resides. When the nerve dies, it disappears and bacteria get into the tunnel, causing an infection. The result is either an acute abscess (very painful), or a chronic infection (sometimes no pain or symptoms at all). Both cause inflammation.

But if the nerve has died, how can it be painful? Teeth sit in bone supported by a ligament. This ligament has an excellent nerve supply, and its nerves will tell you when you have an abscess!

The aim of this treatment is simple to state. "Remove the (dead or dying) nerve from inside the tooth and root, remove or kill any bugs, and fill the space up to stop new bugs from getting in". Easy! (Note that the root remains; it's just the tunnel that is cleaned out).

Most dentists use a series of small files which strip out the inside of the root canal, shaping it in such a way that it can be filled. Most of the time this can be achieved relatively quickly (particularly with modern rotary instruments). A front tooth could easily be prepared and filled in fifteen minutes.

Here's an experiment for you to try. Next time you finish a jar of jam, just get a spoon and see how long it takes to remove all the jam. Just scrape it out and keep going until there's none left. The jar is like the tunnel (the root canal) and the jam is the bacteria and all the nasty stuff they produce. How long did that take you? I'm betting that you gave up before the jar was clean. Well, I'm afraid that's a lot easier than root canal treatment, partly because you can see what you are doing, and partly because glass is a lovely smooth surface, so is easy to clean, right? The inside of a root canal is rough and pitted. The bugs will be hiding in every nook and cranny, and there are often little side tunnels going off the main one which we never manage to get a file into.

Now take your jam jar and run it under the tap. What happens? Most of the jam will disappear. Dentists who can prepare, shape, and fill a root canal quickly are fooling themselves (and you) if they think they have removed even a small proportion of the bugs. The success likelihood of that treatment is tiny. What is the aim of root canal treatment? It's to remove or kill any bugs. So the key is washing it out, over and over again.

We know that we will never wash all the bugs out, so we need to aim to kill the remaining ones. In a hospital, if some blood is spilt on the floor, it's normally covered with bleach and left (typically for fifteen minutes) so the bleach can kill any bugs in the blood spill. The same principle applies to root canal treatment. It takes time for the irrigant (i.e. the liquid we use to wash out the canal) to kill the bugs. A quick root canal treatment without copious washing out is unlikely to achieve its goal.

Which brings me on to another thing, the elephant in the room, if you like: the use of a rubber dam. Now back to your jam jar. You're busy scraping away and washing out, but someone standing beside you is dolloping more jam into the jar. This will affect the likelihood that you will effectively clean it, wouldn't you think? So I am about to upset a significant number of dentists (but they're probably ones who fall into the two categories mentioned earlier, so I don't care if I upset them; they should have followed the warning at the start of the chapter!). The use of a rubber dam when doing root canal treatment is essential. The rubber dam seals off the tooth that is being treated and stops saliva (which is full of bugs) from getting into the tooth. It also allows us to use stronger concentrations of antibacterial irrigant (killing more bugs) as we know the liquid will not be going into your mouth. Root canal treatment is fiddly to do, especially when wearing gloves. Those tiny files we use to get in the canal are not so good if we drop one and you inhale it. The surgery you would need to remove it if it cannot be grabbed and pulled out is not something you would choose to have. A rubber dam eliminates this risk completely.

I am going to make an assumption, but I imagine there is not a specialist in root canal treatment who does not use a rubber dam. I personally would not allow someone to carry out root canal treatment on me without it, and I would not do root canal treatment on a patient without it. So I've opened the flood gates for complaints from members of my profession, but it's more important to me that you are aware of the risks of not having a rubber dam. Sending someone to have surgery on their lung because they have inhaled a file is hardly in keeping with the philosophy I am trying to encourage here!

Now if you have actually done the jam jar experiment, you probably will notice that even with lots of water washing it out and lots of scraping with the spoon, some bits are still left behind. The same is true in root canal treatment. If we do not manage to kill these remaining bugs, they could cause a problem. So the key now is to seal them in to cut off their food source and stop them from growing and reproducing again. There are different techniques available to dentists to achieve this. Many still use the techniques that they used many years ago, but there are better ways now. Additionally the benefit of having a good restoration on top (e.g. a crown) will further help to achieve a seal to cut off the food source.

A tooth that has had unsuccessful root canal treatment will either need to be re-treated or extracted. Otherwise, you will be left with a tooth that has a residual infection, causing inflammation, and we know what that means!

DENTURES

Many people expect a denture to be like their own teeth, and this is almost never the case. Did you know that the chewing force from a denture tooth is probably only about 10% of the force achievable by a natural tooth? (See the previous section on dementia risk and chewing ability for why this is important.) Many denture wearers would like to ignore the fact that they are, to a degree, handicapped. A man with an artificial leg would have great difficulty becoming a professional footballer. The denture wearer must also learn to live with certain limitations. There is a role for dentures, and I find they are successful in many patients but more so when expectations are realistic.

I'll start by being quite frank. Many dentists do not like dentures. Historically people had two main options for a missing tooth: accept the gap or have a denture. In some cases a bridge could be used. Although a denture often helps with chewing, it will be vastly different when compared to natural teeth.

We have a much better alternative with implants. Implants have meant that in almost all cases we can replace teeth with something fixed and firm. There are sometimes medical reasons why we cannot, and sometimes anatomical reasons (e.g. not enough bone) but modern implant techniques have allowed us to overcome many of these. If you have been told in the past you cannot have implants, it's still worth asking again as we can do a lot more nowadays. Normally the reason people choose not to have implants is that they do not want to invest their money in them. That is a shame as the benefit to their mouth, other teeth, and general health is not to be dismissed lightly.

There are nine main features we want to see in a denture:

- We want it to stay in when you talk, laugh, chew, and so on. This is called retention.
- We do not want it to move when you bite. This is the support.
- We do not want it to move from side to side. This is the stability.
- Obviously we want it to look good: the aesthetics.
- We want your speech to be normal: the phonetics.
- We want it to be comfortable and not cause soreness.
- We want it to feel as 'minimally invasive' as possible.
- We want you to be able to chew your food effectively and efficiently.
- We want it to do minimal damage to underlying bone and teeth. (I use the word minimal as it will always cause increased loss of bone, and this can compromise neighbouring teeth.)

Unfortunately these nine features act against each other such that there is ALWAYS some compromise. Let me give two examples. One way to get better retention is with clips, but these compromise the aesthetics. In order for a denture to do minimal damage to supporting bone, it is ideal to cover as much of the jaw bone as possible, but this clearly goes against making it feel 'minimally invasive'.

Our role as clinicians is to try and achieve the best compromise of these features. It is likely that your hopes are not the same as those of your dentist. It is unlikely that your initial thought would be, 'I do not like this denture as it may increase bone loss, meaning that the next denture I have in five to ten years time will be impossible to get on with'. You are more likely to want to achieve one that stays in, looks good, and doesn't feel cumbersome. Our aim would be to provide a denture that aims to achieve as many as possible of the features you would like it have. However, it is IMPOSSIBLE to achieve them all, and I mean in ALL cases.

Many dentures are primarily supported by gums. Gums are not designed for this role and as such do not perform the job very well.

The limitations and problems with dentures are:

- Movement. Dentures are NEVER as firm as teeth are. In other words, the stability is always less than ideal. Please do not expect them to be firm.
- When you bite on a tooth, the force transmits through the root to the ligament, which stretches. The ligament is attached to bone and this pulling force is called a tensile force. This force stimulates bone growth, which is a good thing. When you bite on a denture which rests on the gums, this creates a compressive (i.e. squashing) force. This force causes bone to be resorbed or lost, which is not good.
- Bone loss means the denture will gradually 'sink' over time, so when we try to replace it with a new denture, we find there is less bone to support the new one. You will have adapted your bite gradually to the incorrect position such that it is a real challenge to get your bite back to where it should be. Keeping the bite in the same place that you have become used to will cause even more damage to the underlying bone.
- If you choose to have implants later on, the procedure will be more difficult due to bone loss caused by the dentures.
- Lower full dentures (i.e. when you have no lower teeth) ONLY stay in place if you can train your lips, cheeks, and

tongue to hold them in, or if they have implants to keep them in place

- Lower dentures are notoriously difficult for patients to adapt to. Many never completely adapt to them, and some just cannot tolerate them at all.

- Partial dentures with no natural back teeth are very challenging as the tongue competes for the space where the denture teeth need to be and there is nothing for the dentures to grip against, so they flop about.

- You will get bits of food caught under a denture, which will need cleaning after every meal.

- You may need adhesives to achieve extra retention. Adhesive is unlikely to last all day, so will need replenishing.

- The evidence shows that people with dentures tend to have more plaque in their mouths, which means there are more bugs around to cause that dreaded inflammation, gum disease, and decay.

If you have some of your own teeth, they can help with retention, support, and stability. If you only have a few teeth, they can actually compromise retention, particularly in the upper jaw when there are not enough teeth to keep the denture in place, and the presence of the teeth prevent the denture from forming a seal so it cannot stay up by suction.

Patients often tell us that they know people whose dentures are fine; they can eat steaks and corn on the cob. It is hard to accept that your dentures are unlikely to be this way. The simple reason is that your mouth is different from other people's mouths. The bony support, the 'toughness' of the gums, the saliva, muscle control, and so on, will all play a role, so do not expect the same outcome. One of the major deciding factors is the level of acceptance. Those who accept their dentures and are keen to have them, will have greater success than those who do not want dentures and reluctantly accept them. Many dentists are not keen on dentures because of the damage they do to bone and other teeth and because of their unpredictability, which has nothing to do with clinical expertise, technician's ability, or quality of materials. Implants are a much better alternative.

If you have teeth that need replacing and implants are suitable, I would always recommend implants. They are far superior to dentures and much better for the rest of the health of the mouth and therefore for your general health.

HYGIENIST INPUT/SCALE AND POLISH

It seems that hygienists are a bit like marmite. Either you love 'em or you hate 'em. Some people feel that they have been brushing their own teeth for so many years that they do not need professional input.

I think good hygienists are the unsung heroes helping patients achieve healthy mouths and subsequently better general health. I have seen the mouths of patients who regularly see a great hygienist, and the mouths of those who do not. I can tell you that there is a significant difference. Most of the adult population have some degree of oral inflammation, and hygienists are the best people to help reduce that inflammation. They carry out a combination of procedures including keeping you up to date with the most effective cleaning techniques and tools that are available specifically for your mouth. They help you adapt as your mouth changes (which it will). They also carry out professional cleaning. Even with the best will in the world, most people miss some areas when cleaning. By seeing the hygienist regularly, these areas can be cleaned. This then makes your home regime more effective.

Removal of calculus/tartar is obviously one of the hygienist's roles. If you have a coffee table and you want to make it look nice, you probably spray some polish on it from time to time and give it a shine with a cloth. Let's say I now covered that table in varnish and sprinkled sand into the varnish. When the varnish sets, how effective would your furniture polish be? Calculus is mineral from saliva that sticks to the teeth. If you spend about ten minutes a day cleaning you teeth and gums, that means there are 1430 minutes each day when you are not cleaning (i.e. when I'm sprinkling sand on your table). Is it not surprising that over that time some calculus will collect? Calculus is rough and impossible to clean (like your sandy table!), hence the benefit of regular hygienist care.

I've upset some dentists with my critique of the 'exam'. I've upset some by letting you know that there is a difference in the way restorations can be done. I have upset some by mentioning the rubber dam. So, here's another one of my bugbears. It's the 'exam/scale and polish' (or even worse the 'exam/scrape and polish'). In ten to fifteen minutes the dentist is going to carry out all the checks in the seventeen-point checklist above (in the 'Healthy Mouth Review' section), carry out a thorough professional clean of your mouth, be sure that the technique you are using at the moment to clean at home is still the most appropriate, and show you alternatives as needed? I don't think so. Do you?

Any dental practice that provides the best preventative care possible will offer, as part of its prevention package, regular hygienist care. (It can be carried out by a dentist as long as he or she allows enough time to do it properly.)

HOW OFTEN DO WE NEED TO SEE A HYGIENIST TO ENSURE OUR MOUTHS ARE IN THE BEST CONDITION?

The frequency of visits to the hygienist varies from person to person. However, the time it takes for the bacteria in our mouths to evolve into harmful bacteria (i.e. ones that can lead to bone loss) is about thirteen weeks. This is why people who have had gum disease (which is now stable), or are keen to avoid the diseases in this book will benefit from seeing a hygienist every three months. Those who already suffer from these diseases would be wise to have a hygiene maintenance programme that schedules professional intervention every three months.

DENTAL MEDICINE AND DENTAL TREATMENT

In this book, I have provided a quick rundown of some of the main dental procedures. I hope you can see that there is a difference in how these are performed, and that the difference will have an impact on both the success and longevity of your dental care, your ongoing financial investment in your mouth, and an impact on your general health. Levels of care offered at dental practices vary greatly and so do the fees charged, depending on the level of care. If you feel that your dentist is not offering the best care, you need to either encourage him or her to 'pull his or her socks up' or vote with your feet.

CHAPTER 30

Is There a Benefit in Seeing a Dental Medicine Expert?

Whenever I talk to people or the media about Dental Medicine, and in particular the role of the mouth in influencing general health, they are normally surprised about the mouth's level of influence and about the number of health conditions that are affected. This is true when I talk to members of the public, other dentists, and doctors. I wrote this book as a tool for you to be able to increase your knowledge on this topic, and now is the time to take action.

If we go back in time, and not too long ago, it was normal for dentists to re-use needles. They were disinfected by being put in boiling water for a few minutes. The profession also moved from not wearing gloves, to wearing gloves but re-using them. Fortunately we have moved on from this and use disposable items as much as possible. The thought of going back to this antiquated way of practicing would be unthinkable and unforgivable. Those who do so are quite rightly punished and prevented from working as dentists.[93]

---

93   Daily Mail, 'Disgraced Dentist Who Reused Needles Also Diverted His Patients' Vicodin Prescriptions for His Own Personal Use', *Mail* Online, <http://www.dailymail.co.uk/news/article-2195794/Disgraced-dentist-reused-needles-diverted-patients-Vicodin-prescriptions-personal-use.html>.

Website: http://cnsnews.com/news/article/oklahoma-dental-clinic-inspections-not-necessary

This is just one example of the many changes that occur regularly in the dental field. The dental world must evolve with changes, and I see the philosophy behind Dental Medicine and the way it influences the care we offer as a natural progression for dentistry. Knowing what I do about the impact of oral health on general health, it would be unthinkable for me to go back to practicing 'standard' dentistry. I would not offer the old way to my family and friends, and I believe that patients would not want it either.

A Dental Medicine Expert will already have achieved the level of knowledge and expertise that I would expect a dentist to have. Earlier I introduced the computer-based measuring system that I developed. This can be used to identify which aspects of the mouth are causing inflammation, so we can address the areas of inflammation and help reduce the risk of developing the disease. This tool is made available to Dental Medicine Experts to further improve the care they offer their patients.

If you really want to ensure you receive dental care aimed at improving your general health, you may have to travel a bit further. Obviously this will impact on your time, and only you can choose whether you want to invest that little bit of extra time in reducing the risk of compromising your general health.

You are probably wondering if you will have to pay a lot extra to see a Dental Medicine Expert. There is already a wide range in the fees patients pay for treatment. This is normally a reflection of the quality of the surroundings, the experience of the team providing the care, the materials used, and the expertise of the dentists and the technicians. Does this mean that a Dental Medicine Expert will be expensive? You'll probably find that those who work with this philosophy are charging fees similar to other practices. There will of course be a range of fees, as one would expect. We encourage Dental

Medicine Experts to use high-quality materials with proven track records, and to use technicians who can provide restorations with an excellent fit. We know these higher-quality products are more likely to stand the test of time and so cost less in the long run when compared to something that needs regular replacement. We also know that these high-quality restorations and care will mean there is less likely to be any inflammation, and we have seen how devastating inflammation can be. If you do find that the Dental Medicine Expert's fees are higher than those of other dentists, you will have to choose whether this additional investment in your health and your oral health is right for you. Don't forget good quality treatment that is made to last, and helps your mouth and general health is less likely to need replacement in the future, so saving you money. The initial cost may be higher but the cost effectiveness is much much lower.

CHAPTER 31

How Do I Know if My Dentist Is a Dental Medicine Expert?

I f you have found your dentist's details on www.dentalmedicine. co.uk, you can be sure that he or she has received special training and updates on the subject. You can also be sure that he or she will want to help your mouth be free of inflammation and therefore have a positive effect on your general health.

Other dentists may not be listed on the website, but they may still practice with this philosophy. Perhaps they have studied the literature and have modified the way they work, based on the evidence. You could use this book to quiz them! If your dentist works with this philosophy, perhaps you should point him or her in the direction of www.dentalmedicine.co.uk as he or she may find it of benefit to be a part of our group. I welcome dentists who feel the way I do.

Ask your dentist about some of the things in this book. It is my belief that all dentists should be knowledgeable on all aspects of Dental Medicine. After all, the mouth is the area where we are meant to have the best knowledge, so we should do everything we can to become experts! You need to satisfy yourself that your dentist is up to date on the current research. (Get him or her to buy this book. It will help a lot! Direct your dentist to www.richardguyver.com). If they are not up to date but are prepared to increase their knowledge, I would say this is fine. If they are not prepared to improve their knowledge and therefore their ability to offer you the best care possible, you will need to take that into consideration.

CHAPTER 32

Piecing All the Bits Together

I have offered an extensive look at a number of diseases with proven links to oral health, and some others with possible links. I have also looked briefly at the impact of some diseases on the mouth, and the way we can use the mouth to help us identify diseases. The more research I do around this fascinating subject, the more I want to find out.

When I see a new patient who has not been treated under the philosophy of Dental Medicine, I get a real sense of achievement in knowing that I have helped this patient not only have a healthier mouth and reduced risk of decay, gum disease, oral cancer, and so on, but also a reduced risk of other diseases. When new patients become regular patients, and I see over the years what we have achieved together and how it's still benefitting them, I feel a real sense of pride. After all, that is why I went into dentistry in the first place.

I hope you have found this book useful, and I apologise if it was a bit 'heavy going' in places. Unfortunately this is often the way when dealing with medicine. I wish you good luck on your quest to achieve great health. Just by reading this book, you have put yourself in a much stronger position than many. So, well done on making a great choice! Now is the time to take action and start to take more control of your health. It's time to put some of your new knowledge to good use. I really hope that you do take action, and that you reduce your risk of getting the diseases I have mentioned in this book.

We cannot measure how much longer you will live as a result of what you do now, but be sure to invest some of that extra time in doing great things. Perhaps visit that place you always wanted to go to or help out that charity you always wanted to help. Spend more time with your family and friends and read some books. Maybe even try to mend a broken relationship. After all, there's not much point in living an extra 4006 days if you don't do something with them.

Don't forget that there are additional free resources for readers of this book which can be accessed at www.4006days.com; you will need the following code to access the resources (not case sensitive): hgy4006jujth

CHAPTER 33

Can I Ask a Favour Please?

I spent many hours researching and writing this book. I did this because I am passionate about everyone being able to benefit from the academic research that many great people spend their lives doing. Anyone who has written a book will tell you how much time and effort it takes, challenged by writer's block, and dealing with all the other aspects, such as publication issues, editing, printing, distribution, and so on. I hope you do not mind that I therefore end the book with a request.

I would like all dentists to be Dental Medicine Experts. Then all dental patients would receive this level of care, a level of care that has such a positive impact. To go back to the old way of doing things is, for me, unthinkable. I realise this utopia is a long way off, but I ask you to help me spread the word. Why not lend this book to a friend or colleague, or suggest your friends and colleagues buy their own copy? (Send them to www.richardguyver.com.) When the topic of teeth and mouths comes up, why not inject some of your new-found knowledge into the conversation? You'd be surprised at how interested people are. After all, there are not many people who do not want to live a longer and healthier life. What greater gift can you give to someone than the gift of a longer, healthier life? Time is a resource that we can never replace.

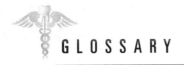

GLOSSARY

ANATOMY (WITH RESPECT TO A TOOTH): the shape and position of a tooth which allows it to function effectively.

AMNIOTIC FLUID: the fluid that surrounds a developing foetus protecting it from pressure.

ANTIOXIDANT: helps reduce the damage caused by sunlight, tobacco, food, and so on.

ARTERIAL: relating to the arteries.

ARTERIES: the blood vessels which carry blood from the heart to the rest of the body.

ATHEROMATOUS (ARTERIAL) DISEASE: the collection of diseases that are caused by the build-up of plaques in the arteries. *see image 10*

BACTERIA: a group of micro-organisms, some of which cause harm to humans.

BETA CELLS (OF THE PANCREAS): the part of the pancreas responsible for releasing insulin.

BICARBONATE: produced in saliva; helps reduce the damage caused by bacteria on teeth.

BISPHOSPHONATES: a type of drug that prevents loss of bone; commonly used to reduce bone loss due to osteoporosis.

BRONCHOSCOPE: a flexible tube with a camera that can be used for removing inhaled objects from the lungs.

BUFFER: When acid affects teeth, a buffer will reduce the impact.

C-REACTIVE PROTEIN: This is normally produced in the liver and is one of the mediators of inflammation.

CARCINOMA: cancer.

CELLS: the basic building blocks of any living organism.

CHRONIC OBSTRUCTIVE PULMONARY DISEASE (COPD): a group of lung diseases including emphysema, chronic bronchitis, and chronic asthma.

COELIAC DISEASE: A disorder of the small intestine in which the sufferer cannot tolerate gluten in the diet. It means other nutrients are not absorbed properly.

COMMUNITY ACQUIRED PNEUMONIA: a form of pneumonia that is 'caught' by people who are not in hospital.

CYTOKINES: part of the immune response that the body releases when subject to injury or disease. Cytokines play a number of different roles including stimulation of blood cell production, and some play a role in immune responses.

DENTAL MEDICINE: the study of the interaction of the mouth on general health and general health on the mouth, and indicators in the mouth about general health. *see image 1*

DERMATOLOGICAL: relating to skin.

DIABETES: a disease in which the cells in the body are not able to 'take in' glucose in the way they should for normal function. This could be due to a reduction in the amount or effectiveness of insulin (required to help them take in the glucose), or a reduction in the response of the cells to insulin (insulin resistance).

DIABETES/DENTAL MATRIX: a measuring tool that dentists can use to identify the impact that the mouth has on diabetes control.

DIGESTION: the process by which our stomach and intestines turn food and drink into smaller components which we need to utilise to carry out our daily functions.

DISCLOSING TABLETS/SOLUTION: brightly coloured dye that can be used in the mouth to show up areas of plaque that have been missed when cleaning.

DNA TEST: DNA is the hereditary material in our cells. Everyone has a different collection of DNA. It's like a fingerprint in the cells in our bodies. A test for DNA is used for many reasons including medical research and forensics.

ENZYMES: These help chemical changes to occur in the body.

GASTRO-INTESTINAL: relating to the oesophagus (food pipe), stomach, and intestines.

GENERAL HEALTH: The diseases and conditions that can affect any part of the body.

GINGIVAL HYPERTROPHY: a condition of the gums, normally related to certain medication which causes the gums to swell and enlarge, making them very difficult to clean.

GINGIVAL CREVICULAR FLUID: a fluid that seeps from the gums around the teeth. In healthy gums it seeps very slowly but speeds up in the presence of inflammation.

GLUCAGON: released by the pancreas when blood sugars are too low (e.g. when exercising); triggers release of glucose stores from the liver.

GLUTEN: a component of wheat, barley, and rye, and several other grains.

GLYCAEMIC CONTROL: The body aims to keep blood glucose at a particular level. In diabetics this function is not carried out very well, so they have to control their own blood sugar with medication or diet (or both). Their ability to do this is their glycaemic control.

HAEMATOLOGICAL: relating to the blood.

HEALTHY MOUTH REVIEW (HMR): the modern-day replacement for a check-up. It involves a thorough assessment of all aspects of the mouth, head, and neck region.

HORMONE: a messenger which travels from one part of the body to influence other parts of the body.

HYPERTENSION: high blood pressure.

IMMUNE COMPONENTS: When the body reacts against injury or disease, it does so by creating an immune response. All the parts of this response are collectively called the immune components.

IMPAIRED FASTING GLUCOSE/IMPAIRED GLUCOSE TOLERANCE/ IMPAIRED GLUCOSE REGULATION/PRE-DIABETES: a condition in which the body shows signs that it is struggling to achieve glycaemic control. The risk of developing diabetes is a lot higher in people with this condition.

INFLAMMATION: the body's response to injury, irritation, or infection.

INSULIN: a hormone released by the pancreas after we eat or drink. It attaches to the cells in the body, allowing those cells to 'take in' the sugar they need in order to function.

INSULIN RESISTANCE: when the cells do not respond normally to insulin; this means that more insulin is needed to achieve the same effect.

INTERPROXIMAL/INTERDENTAL: the area between the teeth.

LICHENOID REACTION: a condition which can affect the skin and the mouth.

LIVER: one of the organs of the body. It has many functions, but in the context of this book, it is involved in producing some inflammatory mediators known as 'acute phase proteins' including C-reactive protein and fibrinogen.

LYMPHADENOPATHY: When there is inflammation, the lymph nodes become enlarged. This can be detected in some areas (e.g. on the neck). The cause can be a simple throat infection, or a sinister thing, such as cancer.

MALIGNANCY: a growth that is cancerous.

MANDIBLE: the lower jaw.

MANDIBULAR: relating to the mandible.

MARKERS: When trying to diagnose certain diseases, we often see if we can detect so-called markers in blood or saliva.

MEDIATORS: The body uses messengers to tell other parts of the body what is happening. These messengers are called mediators and play a very important role in inflammation.

METABOLISM: The body is always taking the things we eat and drink, turning them into useable substances, and disposing of the parts it cannot use. When there is damage, this needs to be repaired. All of these functions are our body's metabolism.

MINERAL: for example, calcium and phosphate. These are the essential substances that our body needs in order to function, grow, and stay healthy.

MYOCARDIAL INFARCT: heart attack.

OBSTRUCTIVE SLEEP APNOEA: See sleep apnoea.

ORAL FLORA: the normal collection of bacteria and fungi in the mouth.

ORAL HEALTH: Oral health can be defined as an absence of disease in the mouth. To achieve oral health, we need to ensure that all the teeth and restorations in the mouth are sound and cleansable, that the patient is able to clean his or her mouth effectively, and that there are no infections present.

OSTEOPOROSIS: a disease that causes increased loss of bone, resulting in brittle bones which are more likely to fracture.

PANCREAS: an organ that sits just behind the stomach. It has a role in digestion and in production of insulin and glucagon.

PERIODONTAL DISEASE: a group of diseases that affect the gums and supporting bone around teeth. It can exist with no detectable signs or very minimal signs. It is rarely painful and can become quite advanced before it is detected. Periodontal disease leads to inflammation, and this inflammation can have an effect on general health. It is one of the major areas of concern in Dental Medicine.

PHARYNGEAL CANCER: cancer of the pharynx which is the area leading back from the mouth (i.e. the throat).

PLAQUE (IN BLOOD VESSELS), ALSO KNOWN AS AN ATHEROMA: a 'thickening' of the wall of a blood vessel. The presence of these reduces the blood flow, and so has an effect on the area of the body supplied by that blood vessel. Pieces can break off and lead to damage, such as a heart attack or a stroke.

PLAQUE (ON TEETH): a collection of bacteria and small fragments of food on teeth. It will cause gum inflammation and can increase the risk of decay, bad breath, and so on.

PLASMA: the fluid part of blood.

PNEUMONIA: lung inflammation caused by bacteria, viruses, or fungi.

PRE-DIABETES/IMPAIRED FASTING GLUCOSE/IMPAIRED GLUCOSE TOLERANCE/IMPAIRED GLUCOSE REGULATION: a condition in which the body shows signs that it is struggling to achieve glycaemic control. The risk of developing diabetes is a lot higher in people with this condition.

PRE-CANCEROUS: a lesion or condition which has a very high chance of becoming cancerous if left.

PRE-ECLAMPSIA: high blood pressure (hypertension) triggered by pregnancy.

PRO-INFLAMMATORY STATE: when there is inflammation that leads to an increase in the number of mediators; if this carries on, the body reaches a pro-inflammatory state and when this occurs, the risk of developing many of the diseases mentioned in this book increases.

PROTEINS: These form the structure of many parts of the body. There are also some mediators that are proteins, as, for example, C-reactive protein.

PSORIASIS: a skin condition in which the body produces excessive tissue which leads to growths. They can cause pain and itchiness.

PYORRHOEA: the old name for periodontal disease.

REMODELLING (WITH RESPECT TO BONE): the process by which bone is removed and replaced by the body to allow it to adapt to change and keep it healthy.

RESTORATIONS: things that dentists place into teeth or the mouth to try and restore the anatomy and function of teeth that have been lost or damaged.

RODENT ULCER: a basal cell carcinoma.

SALIVA: the liquid that is produced in the mouth to aid lubrication and avoid dryness. It helps reduce the risk of decay and inflammation.

SALIVATAN: a part of our saliva which has been shown to increase the release of insulin.

SERUM MARKERS: Doctors try to detect serum markers with blood tests; the presence of serum markers helps diagnose which disease is present.

SJOGREN'S SYNDROME: a condition that causes dryness of the mucous membranes including the eyes and the mouth.

SLEEP APNOEA: a condition in which people completely block their airway in their sleep, leading to periods when they take in no oxygen. It can cause a number of medical problems.

SYSTEMIC DISORDERS: any disease or condition that affects a number of organs or tissues.

TISSUE: a collection of cells which perform a particular function, for example, nerves and skin.

VITAMINS: a group of substances that are required in very small amounts for us to grow and develop.

ABOUT THE AUTHOR

RICHARD GUYVER, BSc, BDS, MFDS, RCSEd, qualified from the prestigious Guys' Hospital Dental School in 2000. He has spent time working in the hospital setting in both maxillofacial surgery and oral medicine departments. He has been working in dental practice for more than ten years and over that time has developed the philosophy behind Dental Medicine. He has founded the Dental Medicine Academy (www.dentalmedicine.co.uk) and the Diabetes and Dentistry Organisation (www.diabetesanddentistry.co.uk). Both organisations are dedicated to raising the awareness of the links between oral and general health, and helping dentists learn how to provide optimal care for their patients.

He is a member of the Royal College of Surgeons of Edinburgh, the Association of Dental Implantology, British Dental Association, British Dental Bleaching Society, and is dental phobia certified.

He has published work on diabetes and its oral health links, and has presented internationally and to the Diabetes Research Network on this topic.

He also presents to 'self-help' groups on the impact of oral health and general health.

Richard is often approached by the media for comment on dental issues, and dental issues related to oral health. His comments/interviews have been published in *Saga Magazine*, the *Daily Mirror*, the *Daily Mail*, *Your Wellness* magazine, and *Maternity & Infant* magazine, to name a few.

Richard is married and has two young sons. He lives on Hayling Island in Hampshire. More information on him and the practices with which he is affiliated can be found at www.richardguyver.com

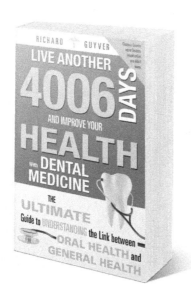

How can you use this book?

MOTIVATE

EDUCATE

THANK

INSPIRE

PROMOTE

CONNECT

Why have a custom version of *Live Another 4006 Days and Improve Your Health with Dental Medicine?*

- Build personal bonds with customers, prospects, employees, donors, and key constituencies

- Develop a long-lasting reminder of your event, milestone, or celebration

- Provide a keepsake that inspires change in behavior and change in lives

- Deliver the ultimate "thank you" gift that remains on coffee tables and bookshelves

- Generate the "wow" factor

Books are thoughtful gifts that provide a genuine sentiment that other promotional items cannot express. They promote employee discussions and interaction, reinforce an event's meaning or location, and they make a lasting impression. Use your book to say "Thank You" and show people that you care.

Live Another 4006 Days and Improve Your Health with Dental Medicine is available in bulk quantities and in customized versions at special discounts for corporate, institutional, and educational purposes. To learn more please contact our Special Sales team at:

1.866.775.1696 • sales@advantageww.com • www.AdvantageSpecialSales.com

Printed in the USA
CPSIA information can be obtained
at www.ICGtesting.com
JSHW012030140824
68134JS00033B/2978